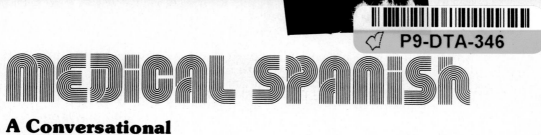

MEDICAL SPANISH

**A Conversational
Approach**

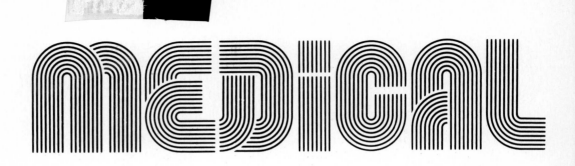

MEDICAL

Maria Antonia Di Lorenzo-Kearon

ST. JOSEPH'S COLLEGE, NEW YORK

ALBERT EINSTEIN COLLEGE OF MEDICINE OF YESHIVA UNIVERSITY

Thomas P. Kearon

ALBERT EINSTEIN COLLEGE OF MEDICINE OF YESHIVA UNIVERSITY

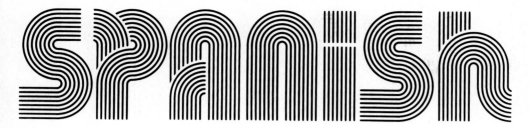

SPANISH

A Conversational Approach

HARCOURT BRACE JOVANOVICH, PUBLISHERS
SAN DIEGO   NEW YORK   CHICAGO   WASHINGTON, D.C.   ATLANTA
LONDON   SYDNEY   TORONTO

To our parents

Anatomical illustrations by Anna Kopczynski

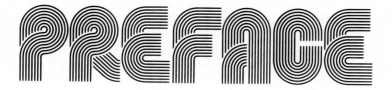
PREFACE

On Labor Day weekend, a highway accident in upstate New York filled a local emergency room with several dozen people in need of immediate assistance. The majority of them were Spanish-speaking tourists who did not understand English. None of the doctors or nurses spoke Spanish. Medical care was therefore severely limited and the patients were subjected to an unusual amount of anguish because they were unable to understand most of what was happening to them.

While this situation was clearly unusual for a hospital in a town in the Northeast, it is not at all uncommon in most of our larger cities and in many rural areas throughout the Southwest. Hispanic Americans are the country's fastest-growing minority, and millions of them still speak little or no English. Adequate medical care can therefore only be provided by members of the health-care professions who speak at least basic Spanish.

Medical Spanish: A Conversational Approach is for students whose primary objective is the development of conversational skills with a specialized vocabulary. Its approach differs from conventional introductions to the language. The basic points of grammar and structure are stated as simply as possible, and, since the emphasis is on ordinary conversation, the grammar has been generally streamlined. The most obvious example of this is the elimination of the second-person singular and plural forms, since the polite forms are generally more appropriate between patients and health-care professionals, and far simpler to learn and use.

The organization of the text stresses continuity. Structures and vocabulary presented in one lesson are regularly drilled and reinforced in subsequent lessons in combination with the new elements. Grammar, structure, and vocabulary are drilled orally by means of substitution, repetition, translation, and directed dialogues. The mini-conversations and dialogues are designed to review grammar and structure, but they also introduce additional vocabulary and idiomatic expressions necessary for the development of proficiency. Emphasis throughout the exercises is not only on the essential medical terms, but on the patient's needs as a human being.

The reading selections are an aid to the development of comprehension skills and introduce additional vocabulary. They also offer possible discussion topics. The role-playing and cued-situation activities call upon the students to use vocabularies and structures to simulate interviews between the patient and the person who is providing health care. The many oral and written exercises are both quickly paced and varied to maintain interest. In conjunction with the other features, these exercises offer the instructor a complete course that can be used in any type of classroom situation. The text can also be easily adapted for home use.

Specialized appendixes summarize the essential information, listing everyday phrases and instructions, verb tenses, and parts of the body (with anatomical diagrams labeled in both languages). The Spanish and English vocabularies include all the words introduced in the text plus other important terms that could be useful in emergency situations.

Perhaps the greatest debt we owe is to the students at Albert Einstein College of Medicine of Yeshiva University, whose questions, insights, and observations helped structure our teaching and this book. We would also like to express our appreciation to Albert Richards, William Dyckes, Anna Kopczynski, Roberta Astroff, and Robert Karpen of Harcourt Brace Jovanovich for their contributions to this book. Special thanks are due to Richard D. Kirschner for his advice and friendship, and to Ronald Cere of the University of Illinois, Urbana, for his constructive suggestions. We are also most grateful to the members of the Department of Community Health of Albert Einstein College of Medicine, especially Elizabeth Williams, for her support and guidance. And finally, our thanks to Craig B. Brush and Lucy Totero of Fordham University, and Albert S. Kuperman of Albert Einstein College of Medicine, for making it all possible.

MARIA ANTONIA DI LORENZO-KEARON

THOMAS P. KEARON

CONTENTS
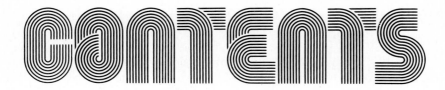

Command forms **108**   Irregular command forms **110**   Conversations:
Physical examinations **112**   Vocabulary: Physical therapy **113**
Dialogue **115**

Vocabulary: Medicines **117**   Present indicative of **dar** **117**
Conversations: **Dar** **119**   Present indicative of **poner** **120**
Conversations: **Poner** **122**   The future tense **123**
Future tense of irregular verbs **124**   Conversations: Future
tense **125**   Dialogue **126**

Preterite tense of regular verbs **128**   Vocabulary: Emergency
situations **131**   Conversations: Preterite tense **132**
Preterite tense of irregular verbs **133**   Conversations:
Preterite tense **136**   Dialogue **137**

Imperfect tense of regular and irregular verbs **140**
Vocabulary: Alcoholism and drug addiction **143**   Contrasting
preterite and imperfect tenses **145**   Conversations:
Alcoholism and drug addiction **146**   Dialogue **148**

Comparison of adjectives **150**   Vocabulary:
Contraception **150**   Conversations: Methods of
contraception **151**   Vocabulary: Pregnancy **153**
Conversations: Past pregnancies **154**   Cued situation:
Medical history and past pregnancies **155**   Conversations:
Present pregnancy **156**   Role playing **156**
Conversations: Labor and delivery **157**   Cued situation:
Labor and delivery **158**   Reading: Pregnancy **159**
Reading: Childbirth **160**   Dialogue **161**

Vocabulary: Postnatal care **164**   Vocabulary: Childhood
ailments and accidents **165**   Vocabulary: Pediatrics **168**
Conversations: Pediatrics **168**   Role Playing **170**   Cued
situation **170**   Dialogue **171**

MEDICAL SPANISH

**A Conversational
Approach**

The alphabet

The Spanish alphabet consists of thirty letters, four more than in English, because **ch, ll, ñ,** and **rr** are used in ways that make it logical to consider them separate letters.

LETTER	NAME	LETTER	NAME	LETTER	NAME
a	a	j	jota	r	ere
b	be	k	ka	rr	erre
c	ce	l	ele	s	ese
ch	che	ll	elle	t	te
d	de	m	eme	u	u
e	e	n	ene	v	ve, uve
f	efe	ñ	eñe	w	doble ve
g	ge	o	o	x	equis
h	hache	p	pe	y	i griega
i	i	q	cu	z	zeta

Pronunciation

VOWELS

As in English, the vowels are **a, e, i, o,** and **u.** The letter **y** is a vowel when it appears as the final letter in a word, as in **soy** (*I am*).

a is similar to the *a* in *father*.
Repeat after your instructor.

1. pa	5. ta	9. papa
2. ca	6. tapa	10. pata
3. ma	7. bata	11. mata
4. ba	8. lata	12. cama

e is similar to the *a* in *cake*, but shorter. There is no diphthongization as in English.

1. pe	5. be	9. teta
2. le	6. nene	10. mate
3. me	7. bebe	11. mesa
4. se	8. vete	12. pesa

i is similar to the *ee* in *see*. Again, it is shorter than the sound in English.

1. li	5. fi	9. pide
2. ti	6. pita	10. cine
3. mi	7. vida	11. casi
4. si	8. mide	12. mima

o is similar to the *o* in *go*. Again, it is not diphthongized. Maintain a clear and open sound.

1. to	5. co	9. moco
2. mo	6. todo	10. codo
3. fo	7. moto	11. pelo
4. so	8. voto	12. palo

u is similar to the *oo* in *boot*.

1. mu	5. bu	9. usa
2. tu	6. pudo	10. supo
3. lu	7. cura	11. tubo
4. su	8. mudo	12. sube

Oral practice

Repeat after your instructor.

1. cama	5. dinero	9. muslo
2. palabra	6. cocina	10. jugo
3. Pedro	7. torso	11. mocoso
4. mesa	8. dormido	12. podoroso

Repeat after your instructor.

1. La mamá habla con el médico.
2. Pedro pela la papa.
3. El brazo está fracturado.
4. La enfermera hace la cama.
5. La cocina está arriba.
6. El hombre usa los músculos para trabajar.
7. No me gusta el jugo.
8. Todos van al hospitál.
9. El médico pone el libro en la mesa.
10. Usted tiene una úlcera.

Stress and accent

For our purposes, *stress* will refer to the greater emphasis that a syllable receives in pronunciation and *accent* to the mark used in Spanish to indicate where the stress goes.

The rule for stress is: if a word ends in a vowel, **n,** or **s,** then the stress is on the next to the last syllable (**vaso, hablan, pesos**); if it ends in a consonant other than **n** or **s,** then the stress is on the last syllable (**comer**). Any deviation from this rule is indicated by an accent (**papá, inglés**).

Syllabification and diphthongs

There are definite rules in Spanish about dividing words into syllables:

1. A word has as many syllables as it has vowels or diphthongs.

2. Each syllable begins with a consonant. For example:

beso	be-so	tomate	to-ma-te
vida	vi-da	lazo	la-zo

3. When there are two consonants together, they are usually separated. For example:

puerta	puer-ta	adelante	a-de-lan-te
perdón	per-dón	excepto	ex-cep-to

   EXCEPTIONS: The following combinations of consonants cannot be broken up: **bl, cl, fl, gl, pl, cr, fr, gr, br, dr,** and **tr.** For example:

madre	ma-dre	palabra	pa-la-bra
mueble	mue-ble	negro	ne-gro

4. An **s** combined with another consonant can never begin a syllable. It must go with the preceeding syllable. For example:

especial	es-pe-cial	estúpido	es-tú-pi-do

5. When there are three consonants in a row, generally, the word is divided after the first consonant (except when the second consonant is an **s**). For example:

hombre	hom-bre	entrar	en-trar
ingle	in-gle	comprendo	com-pren-do

6. In Spanish vowels are considered either strong or weak. The strong vowels are **a, e,** and **o.** The weak vowels are **i** and **u.** When two strong vowels occur together in a word they form two separate syllables. For example:

canoa	ca-no-a	mareado	ma-re-a-do

7. A strong vowel combined with a weak vowel (or two weak vowels together) form only one syllable. For example:

viejo	vie-jo	cuidado	cui-da-do
ejercicio	e-jer-ci-cio	ciudad	ciu-dad

An accent mark indicates that the sound should be broken into two syllables. For example:

tío   tí-o   farmacéutico   far-ma-cé-u-ti-co

8. When two vowels come together in a syllable to form one sound, it is called a diphthong. The following are the diphthongs in Spanish:

ia sounds like *yah* in English: famil**ia**r, f**ia**do, malar**ia**.

ua sounds like *wa* in *wander:* ag**ua**, estat**ua**, enj**ua**gar.

ai sounds like *ie* in *pie:* c**ai**go, p**ai**saje, s**ai**nete.

au sounds like *ou* in *house:* **au**nque, g**au**cho, p**au**sa.

ie sounds like *ye* in *yellow:* c**ie**go, p**ie**l, n**ie**bla.

ue sounds like the word *way:* b**ue**no, d**ue**le, m**ue**la.

ei, ey sounds like the *ay* in h*ay:* p**ei**ne, r**ey**, s**ei**s.

eu has no real equivalent in English. Combine Spanish **e** with **u**: terap**eu**ta, s**eu**dónimo, n**eu**rólogo.

io sounds like the *yo* in *yoga:* rad**io**, secundar**io**, m**io**pe.

uo sounds like *uo* in *quota:* d**uo**décimo, c**uo**ta.

oi, oy sounds like the *oy* in *boy:* b**oi**na, c**oi**to, **oi**go.

ui, uy sounds like the word *we:* c**ui**dado, m**uy**, s**ui**zo.

iu, yu sounds like the word *you:* c**iu**dad, d**iu**rético.

Consonants

b, v	[b]	occurs at the beginning of a breath group or after an **m** or **n**. It sounds like the *b* in *baby:* **b**eso, **v**aso, hom**b**re.
b, v	[ƀ]	occurs in all places except after **m**, **n**, or at the beginning of a breath group. It is similar to [b] except that the lips do not close completely as the sound is made: bo**b**o, to**b**illo, Cu**b**a.
c	[k]	occurs before the vowels **a, o, u,** and all consonants. It is like the *c* in *cat:* **c**omer, **c**asa, se**cc**ión, a**c**tual.
c	[s]	occurs before the vowels **e** and **i.** It is like the *s* in *soap:* **c**eja, **c**ine, co**c**ina.
ch	[ĉ]	sounds like *ch* in *choice* in all places: o**ch**o, ha**ch**a, **ch**aqueta.
d	[d]	occurs after an **n, l,** or at the beginning of a breath group. It is like the *d* in *dark:* **d**iente, an**d**o, fal**d**a.

d	[đ]	occurs in all places except after **n** or **l** or at the beginning of a breath group. It is similar to the *th* in the word *then:* to**d**o, co**d**o, de**d**o.
f	[f]	is identical to the *f* in *fact, effort:* e**f**icaz, **f**laco, **f**rente.
g	[g]	occurs after **n** or at the beginning of a breath group before the letters **a, o,** and **u.** It sounds like the *g* in *gap, globe,* and *angry:* **g**oma, **g**ato, án**g**ulo, **g**uisante, **g**uante.
		NOTE: When **gu** is followed by **e** or **i,** the **u** is not pronounced—unless a diaeresis is placed over the **u** (**güe** or **güi**) to indicate that it is pronounced.
g	[ğ]	occurs before **a, o,** and **u** in all places except after **n** or at the beginning of an utterance. This sound is similar to [g] except that a small amount of air is permitted to pass through the roof of the mouth and the palate, thereby producing a softer sound: a**g**ua, lle**g**a, a**g**otar.
g	[x]	occurs before **e** or **i** and is like the *h* in *hat,* but more guttural: **g**ente, **g**esto, **g**itano.
h		represents no sound in Spanish. It is *always* silent.
j	[x]	is similar to the English *h,* as in *he,* or *wh,* as in *who,* in all places: **j**íbaro, **j**ugo, **j**abón, **j**ota.
l	[l]	similar to the *ll* in si*ll* in all places, except that the tongue strikes farther back on the roof of the mouth, producing a more liquid sound: **l**uz, ca**l**ambre, seña**l**.
ll	[y]	sounds similar to the *y* in *yes* in all places, but the tongue touches the roof of the mouth slightly so that it sounds almost like the *j* in *jelly:* ca**ll**e, meji**ll**a, **ll**evar.
m	[m]	sounds identical to the *m* in *mother* in all places: **m**adre, ca**m**a, enfer**m**o.
n	[n]	sounds the same as the *n* in *noon* in all places: **n**ada, e**n**tre, espi**n**aca.
ñ	[ñ]	sounds like the *ni* in *onion* in all places: se**ñ**or, pu**ñ**o, u**ñ**a, ri**ñó**n.
p	[p]	sounds like the *p* in *paper* in all places, but it is unaspirated, that is, less air is allowed to escape from the lips when the sound is made: **p**apá, **p**luma, **p**lato.
q	[k]	is like the *k* in *kite* in all places. Notice that the **q** is always followed by a **u,** which is not pronounced: **q**ueso, **q**uien, por**q**ue.
r	[r]	occurs in all places except at the beginning of a word, or after **l, n,** or **s.** This sound is called a flap and it is like the *d* in the word *ready* when pronounced rapidly: b**r**azo, na**r**iz, gene**r**al.

rr, r	[r̃]	occurs where the letter **r** follows **n, l,** or **s,** or is at the beginning of a word, and in all places where the letter **rr** occurs. This sound is called a multiple flap or a trill and has no equivalent in the English language: **r**oto, ca**rr**o, en**r**iquecer, al**r**ededor, es **r**ico.
s	[s]	is like the *s* in *stop* or *kiss* in all places: to**s**er, **s**en**s**ación, tri**s**te.
t	[t]	sounds in all places like the *t* in *tip* but it is unaspirated: **t**or**t**a, pa**t**a**t**a, es**t**e.
v		represents the same sound as the letter **b** in all places.
x	[ɡs]	occurs between vowels. It is like the *ggs* in *eggs*: e**x**aminar, e**x**agerar, e**x**asperar, e**x**acto.
		EXCEPTIONS: Mé**x**ico, me**x**icano, are pronounced Méjico, mejicano.
x	[s]	occurs before a consonant. It is the same as the *s* in *stop*: e**x**periencia, e**x**tremo, e**x**ceso.
y	[ɏ]	sounds the same as the letter **ll** in all places: **y**eso, **y**odo, apo**y**ar.
z	[s]	is the same as the *s* in *soap* in all places. It is *never* like the *z* in *zebra:* **z**apato, ta**z**a, **z**ona, feli**z**.

Linking

In a sentence, the final vowel of one word will join with the initial vowel of the next word. Look at the following examples:

Tome‿esta medicina.
Mira‿hacia‿arriba.
Como‿ahora.
Llego‿a las dos.
Como‿en la cafetería.

Oral practice

Pronounce the following sentences keeping in mind the linking of vowels.

1. Me duele el estómago hoy. *My stomach hurts today.*
2. Sigo una dieta estricta. *I am on a strict diet* [*seguir*]
3. La enfermera trabaja en el cuarto. *The nurse is working in the room*
4. El médico examina al paciente. *The doctor is examining the patient.*
5. Me está recetando unas píldoras. *He is prescribing some pills for me.*
6. Mi padre está en el hospital. *My father is in the hospital*
7. La puerta está abierta. *The door is open.*
8. La asistenta hace el trabajo. *The assistant is working.*
9. El hombre está escribiendo una carta. *The man is writing a letter.*
10. Mi madre está bien. *My mother is fine.*

Dialectal variations

Many variations occur in the pronunciation of Spanish. These dialectal differences may be confusing to students who are not familiar with them. The following are guides to variations that may occur in speakers of three major Hispanic groups: Puerto Rican, Mexican, and Cuban. It must be kept in mind that these guides are general and that the variations will not be heard in all speakers from these regions. Also, the same variations may be heard from Spanish-speaking peoples of other geographical areas.

PUERTO RICAN

d is often eliminated at the end of a word: ciudad → ciudá, mitad → mitá.

It is eliminated when intervocalic: hablado → hablao, cuidado → cuidao.

ll is pronounced like the English *j:* inyección → injección, llegar → jegar.

n when it occurs at the end of a word, is pronounced like the *ng* in *singing:* muy bien → muy bieng.

r is pronounced like a **l** when it precedes a consonant: verdad → beldá, puerta → puelta.

When it is at the end of a word, it is also pronounced like an **l**: hablar → hablal, por favor → pol favol.

It is sometimes pronounced like the English *shr* when it is at the beginning of a word: Puerto Rico → Puelto Shrico.

s is eliminated when it precedes a consonant: respirar → repiral, está → etá.

NOTE: Sometimes the entire syllable is eliminated: está bien → tá bieng.

It is eliminated when it comes at the end of a word: ojos azules → ojo azule, los dos → lo dó.

And sometimes it is pronounced like the aspirated *h:* los dos → loh doh.

y is pronounced like the English *j:* yo → jo, yeso → jeso.

Final syllables of words are often eliminated: todo → to, nada → na, para → pa.

Often entire syllables disappear: para abajo → pabajo, para atrás → patrá, para adelante → palante.

MEXICAN

bue, vue is sometimes pronounced as **güe**: bueno → güeno, vuelvo → güelvo.

d is eliminated at the end of a word: usted → usté, pared → paré.

f when followed by **u** sounds like the English *h:* fuerte → huerte, fue → hue.

gua   sounds like the English *wa:* agua → awa, igual → iwal.

gn   often loses the **g**: ignorar → inorar, repugnante → repunante.

ll   sounds like the English **y**: calle → caye, gallina → gayina.

r   before a consonant or at the end of a word often has the sound of **l**: pardo → paldo, hablar → hablal.

CUBAN

c   a hard *c* sound, is often eliminated at the end of a syllable: actor → ator, conductor → condutor.

ch   is pronounced like the English *sh* in *shop:* chico → shico, pecho → pesho.

d   is often eliminated in the combination **-ado**: cerrado → cerrao, cuñado → cuñao.

n   when it occurs at the end of a word, is pronounced like the *ng* in *singing:* saben → sabeng, estación → estacióng.

o   when it occurs at the end of a word, sounds like the English *u* in *lure:* chico → chicu, cuarto → cuartu.

s   often has the sound of the English aspirated *h:* especial → ehpecial, estos → ehtoh. **x** before a consonant has the same sound: extracción → ehtracción.

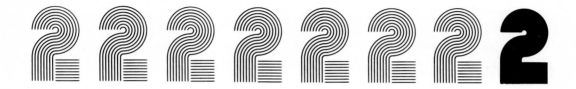

Grammar

PRESENT INDICATIVE OF REGULAR VERBS

A verb is a part of speech that is used to indicate an action or a state of being. Every complete sentence must contain a conjugated verb. In Spanish, there are three types of verbs: one in which the infinitive ends in **-ar** (for example, **hablar**), another that ends in **-er** (**comer**), and a third that ends in **-ir** (**vivir**). The person, number, and tense of verbs are indicated by variations in the endings. Regular verbs have only one stem (the front part of the verb). The tenses of regular verbs are formed by adding the personal endings to this stem.

The present indicative tense in Spanish can be used to show that an action is taking place in the present time (*I am studying Spanish*). It can also be used to express something that takes place in general (*She teaches English*). In addition, the present tense in Spanish may also be used to express an action that will take place in the immediate future (*I'll see you tomorrow*). Thus a typical verb in the present tense, **estudio,** can be translated: *I study, I am studying,* or *I do study.*

FIRST CONJUGATION (-AR VERBS)/*HABLAR*   TO SPEAK

Here is how a regular **-ar** verb, **hablar,** is conjugated in the present tense:

yo	**hablo**	*I speak, am speaking*
él/ella	**habla**	*he/she speaks, is speaking*
usted	**habla**	*you speak, are speaking*
nosotros/nosotras	**hablamos**	*we* (masc./fem.) *speak, are speaking*
ellos/ellas	**hablan**	*they* (masc./fem.) *speak, are speaking*
ustedes	**hablan**	*you* (pl.) *speak, are speaking*

[handwritten margin note: tú ((children) ending: -as]

In normal speech the ending of the verb is often sufficient to indicate who is performing the action. Therefore, the personal pronouns (**yo,** etc.) are sometimes omitted. For example,

Hablo con el médico (*I am speaking with the doctor*). For the sake of clarity, however, it is a good idea to try to use personal pronouns most of the time.

Some regular **-ar** ending verbs are:

aceptar	*to accept*	**necesitar**	*to need*
analizar	*to analyze*	**pasar**	*to enter, happen, pass*
consultar	*to consult*	**preparar**	*to prepare*
curar	*to cure*	**tomar**	*to take* — *to drink alcohol*
doblar	*to bend*	**trabajar**	*to work*
entrar	*to enter*	**usar**	*to use*
estudiar	*to study*	**visitar**	*to visit*

enseñar - to teach

Oral Practice

Answer the questions by following the models.

MODELS:

¿Habla usted con el médico?　　　*Are you speaking with the doctor?*
Sí, yo hablo con el médico.　　　*Yes, I'm speaking with the doctor.*

¿Trabajan ustedes en una clínica?　*Are you (pl.) working in a clinic?*
Sí, nosotros trabajamos en una　　*Yes, we are working in a clinic.*
　clínica.

¿Habla usted con la enfermera (*the female nurse*)?
¿Habla usted con el enfermero (*the male nurse*)?
¿Habla usted con el especialista (*the specialist*)?
¿Habla usted con el terapista (*therapist*)?
¿Habla usted con el farmacéutico (*the pharmacist*)?

¿Acepta usted la decisión (*the decision*)?
¿Acepta usted el dinero (*the money*)?
¿Acepta usted un cheque (*a check*)?
¿Acepta usted el paquete (*the package*)?
¿Acepta usted un regalo (*a gift*)?

¿Trabajan ustedes en la clínica (*the clinic*)?
¿Trabajan ustedes en un hospital (*a hospital*)?
¿Trabajan ustedes en el laboratorio (*the laboratory*)?
¿Trabajan ustedes en la ciudad (*the city*)?
¿Trabajan ustedes en una farmacia (*a pharmacy*)?

¿Entran ustedes en la casa (*the house*)?
¿Entran ustedes en el cuarto (*the room*)?
¿Entran ustedes en la oficina (*the office*)?
¿Entran ustedes en la cocina (*the kitchen*)?
¿Entran ustedes en la sala (*the living room*)?

MODELS:

¿Habla él con el médico?
Sí, él habla con el médico.

Is he speaking with the doctor?
Yes, he is speaking with the doctor.

¿Hablan ellas con el médico?
Sí, ellas hablan con el médico.

Are they (fem.) *speaking with the doctor?*
Yes, they're speaking with the doctor.

¿Estudia él el español (*Spanish*)?
¿Estudia ella la medicina (*medicine*)?
¿Estudia él la biología (*biology*)?
¿Estudia ella el inglés (*English*)?
¿Estudia él la anatomía (*anatomy*)?

¿Consulta ella con la doctora (*female doctor*)?
¿Consulta él con el anestesiólogo (*anesthesiologist*)?
¿Consulta ella con la paciente (*female patient*)?
¿Consulta él con el paciente (*male patient*)?
¿Consulta ella con el técnico (*technician*)?

¿Enseñan ellos la medicina (*medicine*)?
¿Enseñan ellas la lección (*the lesson*)?
¿Enseñan ellos la biología (*biology*)?
¿Enseñan ellas el español (*Spanish*)?
¿Enseñan ellos el inglés (*English*)?

Grammar

GENDER OF NOUNS AND ARTICLES, PLURALIZATION OF NOUNS

GENDER OF NOUNS AND ARTICLES: In Spanish all nouns are either masculine or feminine. Generally, nouns ending in **-o** or which refer to male beings are masculine. Nouns ending in **-a** or which refer to female beings are feminine. There are exceptions, however. The word **día** (*day*), for instance, is a masculine noun although it ends in **-a.** Another exception is the word **mano** (*hand*), which is a feminine noun.

The definite article used before a masculine singular noun is **el** (*the*); the indefinite article is **un** (*a, an*). The definite article used before a feminine singular noun is **la,** the indefinite article is **una.**

Generally, nouns ending in **-ador, -al, -ente, -ma,** and **-or** are masculine. Nouns ending in **-ción, -sión, -dad, -tad,** and **-ud** are usually feminine. Some nouns ending in **-a** can be either masculine or feminine. Their gender is indicated by the use of the definite article. For example: **el** or **la terapista,** the therapist; **el** or **la especialista,** the specialist.

PLURALIZATION: Nouns that end in a vowel form the plural by adding **-s.** Nouns ending in a consonant form the plural by adding **-es.** The definite articles **el** and **la** become **los** and **las** respectively when they accompany plural nouns. The indefinite articles **un** and **una** become **unos** and **unas** (*some* or *a few*).

Oral practice

Change the italicized nouns by following the model.

MODEL:

Hablo con el médico. I'm speaking with the doctor.
Hablo con los médicos. I'm speaking with the doctors.

1. Hablamos con *la enfermera.* *We are speaking ī the nurse*
2. Trabajo en *la clínica.* *I work in the clinic.*
3. Consultan con *el especialista.* *They are consulting the specialist*
4. Aceptamos *el regalo.* *We are accepting the gift.*
5. El médico entra en *la casa.* *The doctor is entering in the house.*
6. Entro en *el hospital.* *I am entering in the hospital.*
7. La enfermera consulta con *el terapista.* *The nurse is consulting ī the therapist.*
8. La doctora analiza *el problema.* *The doctor is analyzing the problema.*
9. Aceptamos *el cheque.* *We are accepting the check.*
10. Hablan con *el farmacéutico.* *They are speaking ī the pharmacist.*

MODEL

Hablo con los médicos. I'm speaking with the doctors.
Hablo con el médico. I'm speaking with the doctor.

1. Trabajamos con *las enfermeras.* *We are working ī some nurses.*
2. Consulto con *unas doctoras.* (a) (some) *I am consulting ī some doctors (female).*
3. Aceptan *las decisiones.* *They are accepting the decisions.*
4. Enseña *unas lecciones.* *He is teaching some lessons.*
5. Hablo con *los terapistas.* *I am speaking ī the therapists.*
6. Consultamos con *unos técnicos.* *We are consulting ī some technicians.*
7. Entramos en *las farmacias.* *We are entering the pharmacy.*
8. Necesitan *unos paquetes.* *They need some packages.*
9. Entran en *las salas.* *They are entering the rooms.*
10. Visito *unas ciudades.* *I am visiting some cities.*

SECOND CONJUGATION (-ER VERBS)/*COMER* TO EAT

yo	**com<u>o</u>**	I eat
él/ella	**com<u>e</u>**	he/she eats
usted	**com<u>e</u>**	you eat
nosotros/nosotras	**comemos**	we eat
ellos/ellas	**comen**	they eat
ustedes	**comen**	you (pl.) eat

Some other regular **-er** ending verbs are:

aprender	to learn	**correr**	to run
beber	to drink	**responder**	to answer
comprender	to understand	**vender**	to sell

Grammar

NEGATIVES

In Spanish a sentence is made negative by placing the word **no** before the verb. In answering questions, one often begins the sentence with an additional **no** for emphasis, in much the same way as is done in English. For example:

¿Toma Ud. la medicina?　　　　　*Are you taking the medicine?*
No, yo no tomo la medicina.　　　*No, I'm not taking the medicine.*

Unlike English, Spanish uses the double negative.

¿Toma usted algo para el dolor?　　*Are you taking anything for the pain?*
No, yo no tomo nada.　　　　　　*No, I'm not taking anything (nothing).*

Oral practice

Answer the questions with two responses following the model.

MODEL:

¿Bebe usted el jugo?　　　　　　*Are you drinking the juice?*
No, yo no bebo el jugo.　　　　　*No, I'm not drinking the juice.*
No, yo no bebo nada.　　　　　　*No, I'm not drinking anything.*

¿Bebe usted el líquido (*liquid*)?
¿Bebe usted la cerveza (*beer*)?
¿Bebe usted el vino (*wine*)?
¿Bebe usted la leche (*milk*)?
*¿Bebe usted el agua (*water*)?

¿Comprenden ustedes la lección (*lesson*)?　　*No, nosotros no compredemos —*
¿Comprenden ustedes la pregunta (*question*)?　*No, nosotros no compredemos nada.*
¿Comprenden ustedes el idioma (*language*)?
¿Comprenden ustedes la idea (*idea*)?
¿Comprenden ustedes la explicación (*explanation*)?

¿Vende ella la casa (*house*)?
¿Vende ella el café (*coffee*)?
¿Vende ella el té (*tea*)?
¿Vende ella los libros (*books*)?
¿Vende ella la medicina (*medicine*)?

* The word **agua** (*water*) is a feminine noun but uses the masculine definite article when it is in the singular form because of the similarity of the vowels in each word. Use the feminine definite article when the word is pluralized— **las aguas.**

¿Responden ellos a la pregunta (*question*)?
*¿Responden ellos a la pregunta del hombre (*man's question*)?
¿Responden ellos a la pregunta de la mujer (*woman's question*)?
¿Responden ellos a la llamada telefónica (*phone call*)?
*¿Responden ellos al timbre (*bell*)?

THIRD CONJUGATION (-IR VERBS)/*VIVIR*   TO LIVE

yo	**vivo**	*I live*
él/ella	**vive**	*he/she lives*
usted	**vive**	*you live*
nosotros/nosotras	**vivimos**	*we live*
ellos/ellas	**viven**	*they live*
ustedes	**viven**	*you* (pl.) *live*

Some other regular **-ir** ending verbs are:

abrir	*to open*
decidir	*to decide*
escribir	*to write*
recibir	*to receive*
sufrir	*to suffer*

Oral practice

Answer the questions in the affirmative following the model.

¿Vive usted en la casa?   *Are you living in the house?*
Sí, yo vivo en la casa.   *Yes, I am living in the house.*

¿Abre usted la puerta (*door*)?   *Si, yo abro* ____
¿Abre usted la ventana (*window*)?
¿Abre usted la caja (*box*)?
¿Abre usted la botella (*bottle*)?
¿Abre usted el libro (*book*)?

¿Escribe él la carta (*letter*)?   *Si, el escribe* ____
¿Escribe él el libro (*book*)?
¿Escribe él la receta (*prescription*)?
¿Escribe él la dirección (*address*)?
¿Escribe él la lista (*list*)?

¿Reciben ustedes el dinero (*money*)?   *Si, nosotros recibimos* ____
¿Reciben ustedes la comida (*food*)?

---

* Whenever the preposition **de,** meaning *of, from,* immediately precedes the definite article **el,** the two words combine to form the contraction **del.** The preposition **a,** meaning *to,* combines with the definite article **el** to form the contraction **al.**

¿Reciben ustedes el regalo (*gift*)?
¿Reciben ustedes las noticias (*news*)?
¿Reciben ustedes los resultados (*results*)?

¿Sufren ellas de dolores de cabeza (*headaches*)?
¿Sufren ellas de dolores del estómago (*stomach*)?
¿Sufren ellas de tos (*cough*)?
¿Sufren ellas de los nervios (*nerves*)?
¿Sufren ellas de catarros frecuentes (*frequent colds*)?

Grammar

WORD ORDER

In a declarative sentence in Spanish, the subject comes first, followed by the verb, and then the object. In an interrogative sentence, the verb is placed before the subject and question marks are put at the beginning and the end of the sentence.

DECLARATIVE: **El niño bebe el jugo.** *The child is drinking the juice.*

INTERROGATIVE: **¿Bebe el niño el jugo?** *Is the child drinking the juice?*

Oral practice

Change these declarative sentences into interrogative sentences.

1. El enfermero habla español. *¿Habla español el enfermero?*
2. El paciente abre una puerta. *¿Abre una puerte el paciente?*
3. La doctora entra en el cuarto. *¿Entra en el cuarto la doctora?*
4. La mujer bebe un líquido. *¿Bebe un líquido la mujer?*
5. El hombre comprende la lección. *¿Comprende la lección el hombre?*
6. El farmacéutico trabaja en la clínica. *¿Trabaja en la clínica el farmacéutico?*
7. Ella consulta con unos especialistas. *¿Consulta ella con unos especialistas?*
8. Ellos escriben la dirección. *¿Escriben ellos la dirección?*
9. El paciente sufre de tos. *¿Sufre el paciente de tos?*
10. Nosotros escribimos la carta. *¿Escribimos nosotros la carta?*

Grammar

PRESENT INDICATIVE OF THE IRREGULAR VERB *TENER* (TO HAVE)

Irregular verbs differ from regular verbs in that they have changes either in their stems or in their endings.

yo	**tengo**	*I have*
él/ella	**tiene**	*he/she has*
usted	**tiene**	*you have*

nosotros/nosotras	**tenemos**	*we have*
ellos/ellas	**tienen**	*they have*
ustedes	**tienen**	*you* (pl.) *have*

Oral practice

Answer the sentences first in the affirmative and then in the negative.

MODEL:

¿Tiene usted tos?	*Do you have a cough?*
Sí, yo tengo tos.	*Yes, I have a cough.*
No, yo no tengo tos.	*No, I don't have a cough.*

1. ¿Tiene usted problemas?
2. ¿Tiene usted dolor del estómago?
3. ¿Tiene usted dolor de cabeza?
4. ¿Tiene usted dinero?
5. ¿Tiene usted catarro?

Change the subjects and the verbs to the plural.

| **El paciente tiene tos.** | *The patient has a cough.* |
| **Los pacientes tienen tos.** | *The patients have a cough.* |

1. El hombre tiene dolor.
2. La mujer tiene problemas.
3. La paciente tiene tos.
4. Tengo dolor de cabeza.
5. Ella tiene catarro.

Grammar

EXPRESSIONS WITH *TENER*

Although it means *to have,* the verb **tener** is used to express a number of things that are expressed by the verb *to be* in English.

tener calor	*to be warm*	**tener prisa**	*to be in a hurry*
tener frío	*to be cold*	**tener razón**	*to be right*
tener hambre	*to be hungry*	**no tener razón**	*to be wrong*
tener miedo	*to be afraid*	**tener sed**	*to be thirsty*
tener paciencia	*to be patient*	**tener sueño**	*to be sleepy*

Oral practice

Answer the questions using the cues.

MODEL:

¿Quién tiene calor?	*Who is warm?*
● **la señora García**	*● Mrs. García*
La señora García tiene calor.	*Mrs. García is warm.*

1. ¿Quién tiene calor?
   ● la enfermera   ● el paciente   ● las doctoras   ● usted   ● ellos

2. ¿Quién tiene frío?
   ● nosotros   ● el hombre   ● los pacientes   ● la señora Menéndez   ● yo

3. ¿Quién no tiene razón?
   ● ellas   ● los hombres   ● nosotras   ● los médicos   ● el farmacéutico

4. ¿Qué tiene el paciente?
   ● sed   ● sueño   ● miedo   ● prisa   ● hambre

5. ¿Qué tienen los médicos?
   ● paciencia   ● hambre   ● sed   ● razón   ● prisa

Grammar

TENER QUE

The Spanish expression **tener que** corresponds to the English *to have to*. Since there is no verb that corresponds exactly to the English word *must*, this construction and several like it are quite frequently used. For example:

El señor Gómez tiene que hablar con	*Mr. Gómez has to speak with a doctor.*
el médico.	

Oral practice

Change the sentences to the plural by following the model.

Yo tengo que hablar con la	*I must speak with the nurse.*
enfermera.	
Nosotros tenemos que hablar con las	*We must speak with the nurses.*
enfermeras.	

1. El hombre tiene que hablar con un terapista.
2. La enfermera tiene que consultar con el paciente.
3. El terapista tiene que trabajar en la clínica.

4. El especialista tiene que responder a la pregunta del paciente.
5. Ella tiene que vender la casa al hombre.
6. Tengo que escribir la carta a la mujer.
7. Él tiene que abrir la ventana de la sala.
8. El médico tiene que escribir una carta.
9. Tengo que aceptar el regalo.
10. Ella tiene que comprar el libro.

Written practice

Translate into English.

1. El especialista trabaja en un hospital. *The specialist is working in a hospital.*
2. El farmacéutico prepara la receta en la farmacia. *The pharmacist is preparing the prescription in the pharmacy.*
3. El paciente no acepta la decisión del médico. *The patient is not accepting the decision of the doctor.*
4. El hombre corre al hospital. *The man is running to the hospital.*
5. Bebemos el café. *We are drinking the coffee*
6. No tengo que tomar la medicina. *I don't have to take the medicine.*
7. El médico tiene que escribir una receta. *The doctor has to write the prescription*
8. Los hombres abren las ventanas. *The men are opening the windows.*
9. La enfermera tiene calor. *The nurse is warm.*
10. La paciente tiene hambre. *The patient is hungry.*

Translate into Spanish.

1. I have to take the pills. *Yo tengo que tomar los píldoras.*
2. The patient (*masc.*) is drinking the juice. *El paciente bebe el jugo.*
3. The pharmacist works in a clinic. *El farmacéutico trabaja en una clínica.*
4. We (*fem.*) don't understand the question. *Nosotras no comprendemos la pregunta.*
5. The patient (*fem.*) is suffering. *La paciente sufre.*
6. The woman is cold. *La mujer tiene frío.*
7. The therapist is entering the room. *El terapista entra la cuarta.*
8. I must speak with the patient (*masc.*) *Yo tengo que hablar con el paciente.*
9. He has to work in the hospital. *El tengo que trabajar en el hospital.*
10. The doctors are hungry. *Los doctors tiene hambre.*

Dialogue

PACIENTE: Buenas tardes, doctor.
MÉDICO: Buenas tardes. ¿Habla usted inglés?
PACIENTE: No, no hablo inglés.
MÉDICO: ¿Qué tiene usted?
PACIENTE: Tengo (un) dolor de cabeza muy fuerte.
MÉDICO: ¿Qué toma usted para el dolor de cabeza?
PACIENTE: No tomo nada.

MÉDICO: Usted sufre de los nervios. Tiene que tomar las pastillas que *le* receto (para usted) y descansar mucho.

PACIENTE: Muchas gracias, doctor.

MÉDICO: De nada. Usted tiene que regresar en una semana.

PACIENTE: Muy bien, doctor. Adiós.

VOCABULARY

Buenas tardes.   *Good afternoon.*

el dolor de cabeza   *headache*

muy   *very*

fuerte   *strong*

para   *for*

nada   *nothing*

sufrir de   *to suffer from*

los nervios   *nerves*

la pastilla } *pill – most common*
la píldora
el comprimido – compound

recetar   *to prescribe*

descansar   *to rest*

mucho   *much, a lot*

Muchas gracias.   *Thank you very much.*

De nada.   *You're welcome.*

regresar   *to return*   *volver – to return*

la semana   *week*

Muy bien.   *very well*

Adiós.   *Goodbye.*

PATIENT: Good afternoon, doctor.

DOCTOR: Good afternoon. Do you speak English?

PATIENT: No, I don't speak English.

DOCTOR: What is wrong?

PATIENT: I have a very bad headache.

DOCTOR: What are you taking for the headache?

PATIENT: I'm not taking anything.

DOCTOR: You are suffering from nervousness. You must take the pills which I'm prescribing and rest a lot.

PATIENT: Thank you very much, doctor.

DOCTOR: You're welcome. You must return in a week.

PATIENT: Very well, doctor. Goodbye.

QUESTIONS ON DIALOGUE

1. ¿Habla el paciente inglés?
2. ¿Qué tiene el paciente?
3. ¿Qué toma el paciente para el dolor?
4. ¿De qué sufre el paciente?
5. ¿Qué tiene que tomar el paciente?
6. ¿Tiene que descansar mucho el paciente?
7. ¿Tiene que regresar el paciente?

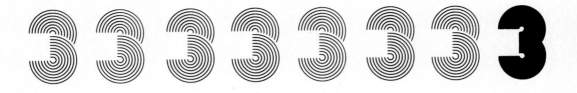

Grammar

PRESENT INDICATIVE OF THE IRREGULAR VERB *SER* (TO BE)

yo	**soy**	*I am*
él/ella	**es**	*he/she is*
usted	**es**	*you are*
nosotros/nosotras	**somos**	*we are*
ellos/ellas	**son**	*they are*
ustedes	**son**	*you* (pl.) *are*

There are two different verbs in Spanish for the English verb *to be*. The first one that we will study is **ser,** which is used to express more permanent or inherent qualities, such as a person's profession. For example:

El hombre es médico.　　　　　　　*The man is a doctor.*

Note that this verb does not require the use of an indefinite article before the noun. The indefinite article is only used when the noun is modified by an adjective:

El hombre es un médico famoso.　　*The man is a famous doctor.*

Oral practice

Answer the questions by following the model.

　***¿Es Ud. abogado?**　　　　　　*Are you a lawyer?*
　Sí, soy abogado.　　　　　　　*Yes, I'm a lawyer.*

* The abbreviated forms for **usted (Ud.)** and **ustedes (Uds.)** will be used from here on.

1. ¿Es Ud. actor (*actor*)?
2. ¿Es Ud. actriz (*actress*)?
3. ¿Es Ud. ama de casa (*housewife*)?
4. ¿Es Ud. artista (*artist*)?
5. ¿Es Ud. atleta (*athlete*)?
6. ¿Es Ud. autor(-a) (*author*)?
7. ¿Es Ud. barbero (*barber*)?
8. ¿Es Ud. bombero (*fireman*)?
9. ¿Es Ud. cajero(-a) (*cashier*)?
10. ¿Es Ud. camarero(-a) (*waiter, waitress*)?
11. ¿Es Ud. carnicero (*butcher*)?
12. ¿Es Ud. carpintero (*carpenter*)?
13. ¿Es Ud. cartero (*mailman*)?
14. ¿Es Ud. conductor de ambulancia (*ambulance driver*)?
15. ¿Es Ud. dependiente(-a) (*clerk*)?
16. ¿Es Ud. electricista (*electrician*)?
17. ¿Es Ud. hombre de negocios (*businessman*)?
18. ¿Es Ud. ingeniero(-a) (*engineer*)?
19. ¿Es Ud. maestro(-a) (*teacher*)?
20. ¿Es Ud. mecánico (*mechanic*)?
21. ¿Es Ud. mujer de negocios (*businesswoman*)?
22. ¿Es Ud. policía (*policeman, policewoman*)?
23. ¿Es Ud. profesor(-a) (*professor*)?
24. ¿Es Ud. recepcionista (*receptionist*)?
25. ¿Es Ud. secretario(-a) (*secretary*)?

Grammar

ADJECTIVES

Adjectives are parts of speech that limit or describe nouns or pronouns. They must agree in gender and number with the nouns or pronouns that they describe. If an adjective ends in an **-o,** its feminine form ends in an **-a.** Some adjectives end in **e** for both the masculine and feminine forms. In all cases, the plural is formed by adding an **-s.** Descriptive adjectives usually follow the nouns that they modify. For example:

una muchacha bonita	*a pretty girl*
el hombre famoso	*the famous man*
un especialista importante	*an important specialist*
unas mujeres competentes	*some competent women*

The verb **ser** is not used with all adjectives, but principally with those that describe more permanent or inherent qualities, such as a person's physical traits and personality.

Oral practice

The following questions combine the verb **ser** with a number of basic adjectives that describe physical traits and personality. Answer the questions by following the models. Make sure that the adjectives agree in gender and number with the nouns that they describe.

¿Es simpático el actor?	*Is the actor pleasant?*
Sí, es un actor simpático.	*Yes, he is a pleasant actor.*
¿Es hermosa la actriz?	*Is the actress beautiful?*
Sí, es una actriz hermosa.	*Yes, she is a beautiful actress.*

1. ¿Es alto (*tall*) el bombero?
2. ¿Es bajo (*short*) el cartero?
3. ¿Es delgada (*slender*) la camarera?
4. ¿Es flaca (*thin, skinny*) la actriz?
5. ¿Es gordo (*fat*) el carnicero?
6. ¿Es guapo (*good-looking*) el maestro?
7. ¿Es linda (*pretty*) la secretaria?
8. ¿Es feo (*ugly*) el atleta?
9. ¿Es buena (*good*) la maestra?
10. ¿Es malo (*bad*) el artista?
11. ¿Es simpática (*nice, pleasant*) la autora?
12. ¿Es antipático (*unpleasant, disagreeable*) el barbero?

Answer the questions in the affirmative by following the model.

¿Son fuertes los hombres?	*Are the men strong?*
Sí, los hombres son fuertes.	*Yes, the men are strong.*

1. ¿Son importantes (*important*) los profesores?
2. ¿Son pacientes (*patient*) las amas de casa?
3. ¿Son impacientes (*impatient*) las actrices?
4. ¿Son sensibles (*sensitive*) los artistas?
5. ¿Son insensibles (*insensitive*) los actores?
6. ¿Son inteligentes (*intelligent*) las maestras?
7. ¿Son competentes (*competent*) las secretarias?
8. ¿Son incompetentes (*incompetent*) los electricistas?
9. ¿Son valientes (*brave*) los bomberos?
10. ¿Son diligentes (*diligent*) los secretarios?
11. ¿Son agradables (*pleasant*) los carteros?
12. ¿Son desagradables (*unpleasant*) los mecánicos?

Change the sentences using the cues.

Las camareras son flacas.	*The waitresses are thin.*
• **el camarero**	*• the waiter*
El camarero es flaco.	*The waiter is thin.*

1. El maestro es antipático.
2. Los abogados son competentes.
3. La policía es paciente.
4. El conductor de ambulancia es valiente.
5. Los hombres de negocios son simpáticos.
6. La secretaria es guapa.
7. Los ingenieros son inflexibles.
8. Las profesoras son impacientes.
9. La atleta es diligente.
10. El cajero es incompetente.

- las maestras
- la abogada
- el policía
- la conductora de ambulancia
- la mujer de negocios
- el secretario
- las ingenieras
- el profesor
- los atletas
- las cajeras

Answer the questions in the affirmative using the English cues.

¿Cómo es el médico?
El médico es agradable.

What is the doctor like?
The doctor is pleasant.

1. ¿Cómo es el cardiólogo (*cardiologist*)?
2. ¿Cómo es el dentista (*dentist*)?
3. ¿Cómo es el ginecólogo (*gynecologist*)?
4. ¿Cómo es el neurólogo (*neurologist*)?
5. ¿Cómo es el oftalmólogo (*opthalmologist*)?
6. ¿Cómo es el óptico (*optician*)?
7. ¿Cómo es el ortopédico (*orthopedic*)?
8. ¿Cómo es el pediatra (*pediatrician*)?
9. ¿Cómo es el psicólogo (*psychologist*)?
10. ¿Cómo es el psiquíatra (*psychiatrist*)?

- patient
- nice
- impertinent
- intelligent
- inflexible
- disagreeable
- impatient
- competent
- flexible
- diligent

Conversations

A: ¿En qué trabaja Ud.?
B: Soy camarero.
A: ¿Es un trabajo duro?
B: Sí, es un trabajo duro.
A: ¿Por qué?
B: Porque tengo que trabajar muchas horas.

A: What do you do?
B: I'm a waiter.
A: Is it hard work?
B: Yes, it's hard work.
A: Why?
B: Because I have to work many hours.

A: ¿Qué trabajo hace Ud.?
B: Soy cartero.
A: ¿Es un empleo exigente?
B: Sí, es muy exigente.
A: ¿Por qué es exigente?
B: Porque tengo que caminar mucho.

A: What work do you do?
B: I'm a mailman.
A: Is it a demanding job?
B: Yes, it's very demanding.
A: Why is it demanding?
B: Because I have to walk a lot.

A: ¿Tiene trabajo?
B: Sí, soy bombero.

A: Are you employed?
B: Yes, I'm a fireman.

A: ¿Es un trabajo difícil?

B: Sí, es difícil y es peligroso también.

A: ¿Por qué es peligroso?

B: Porque tengo que inhalar humos y
    subir escaleras.

A: Is it a difficult job?

B: Yes, it's difficult and it is dangerous
    also.

A: Why is it dangerous?

B: Because I have to inhale fumes and
    climb stairs.

Grammar

POSSESSIVE ADJECTIVES

The possessive adjectives are:

SINGULAR	PLURAL	
mi	**mis**	*my*
su	**sus**	*your, his, her, its, their*
nuestro	**nuestros**	*our* (masc.)
nuestra	**nuestras**	*our* (fem.)

The possessive adjectives **mi, mis** and **su, sus** must agree in number with the noun they modify.

Mi padre es médico.	*My father is a doctor.*
Mis padres son médicos.	*My parents are doctors.*

The possessive adjective **nuestro, -a, -os, -as** must agree with the noun it modifies in both number and gender.

Nuestra madre es doctora.	*Our mother is a doctor.*
Nuestras madres son doctoras.	*Our mothers are doctors.*

Su or **sus** can mean *your, his, her, its,* or *their.* If the meaning is not clear from the context, it can be clarified by using **de él, de ella, de Ud., de ellos, de ellas,** or **de Uds.** instead of the possessive adjective.

Su padre es médico.	*His/her/your/their father is a doctor.*
El padre de ella es médico.	*Her father is a doctor.*

Oral practice

Answer the questions in the affirmative by following the model.

¿Es médico su padre?	*Is your father a doctor?*
Sí, mi padre es médico.	*Yes, my father is a doctor.*

1. ¿Es enfermero su hijo (*son*)?
2. ¿Es enfermera su hija (*daughter*)?
3. ¿Es bombero su hermano (*brother*)?

4. ¿Son profesoras sus hermanas (*sisters*)?
5. ¿Son cardiólogos sus primos (*male cousins*)?
6. ¿Son amas de casa sus primas (*female cousins*)?
7. ¿Es barbero su sobrino (*nephew*)?
8. ¿Es artista su sobrina (*niece*)?
9. ¿Son autores sus tíos (*uncles*)?
10. ¿Es camarera su tía (*aunt*)?
11. ¿Es dentista su cuñado (*brother-in-law*)?
12. ¿Es atleta su cuñada (*sister-in-law*)?
13. ¿Es ginecólogo su suegro (*father-in-law*)?
14. ¿Es pediatra su suegra (*mother-in-law*)?
15. ¿Es óptico su yerno (*son-in-law*)?
16. ¿Son psiquiatras sus nueras (*daughters-in-law*)?
17. ¿Es psicólogo su abuelo (*grandfather*)?
18. ¿Es abogada su abuela (*grandmother*)?
19. ¿Es ingeniero su nieto (*grandson*)?
20. ¿Es policía su nieta (*granddaughter*)?
21. ¿Es carnicero su esposo (*husband*)?
22. ¿Es recepcionista su esposa (*wife*)?
23. ¿Es actor su marido (*husband*)?
24. ¿Es profesora su mujer (*wife*)?

Grammar

MORE USES OF THE VERB *SER*

Another way in which **ser** is used is to refer to a person's nationality or place of origin. For example:

Juan es de Colombia.   *Juan is from Colombia.*

Oral practice

Answer the questions with complete sentences using the cues.

¿De dónde es Juan?   *Where is Juan from?*
Juan es de los Estados Unidos.   *Juan is from the United States.*

1. ¿De dónde es el médico?
2. ¿De dónde es el paciente?
3. ¿De dónde es su padre?
4. ¿De dónde es la enfermera?
5. ¿De dónde es su hermano?
6. ¿De dónde son sus padres?
7. ¿De dónde son Uds.?

- los Estados Unidos
- Colombia
- Puerto Rico
- la República Dominicana
- México
- Venezuela
- el Panamá

8. ¿De dónde son sus primos?
9. ¿De dónde es Ud.?
10. ¿De dónde es el señor Martínez?

- España
- Cuba
- el Ecuador

Written practice

Translate the sentences into Spanish.

1. He is a famous doctor.
2. My father is a pleasant man.
3. She is very nice.
4. My mother is from Spain.
5. The nurses in the hospital are very friendly.
6. The patient is from Puerto Rico.
7. I'm a mechanic.
8. Our doctor is short.
9. My sister is tall.
10. His uncle is from Cuba.
11. She is very intelligent.
12. The woman doesn't speak English.
13. My job is very demanding.
14. The technician is very handsome.
15. The work is difficult.

Conversations

A: ¿Tiene Ud. una familia grande?
B: Sí, tengo una familia grande.
A: ¿Quiénes son los miembros de su familia?
B: Tengo dos hijos y tres hijas.
A: ¿Hay otros que viven en su casa?

B: Sí, la abuela de mi esposa vive con nosotros.

A: Do you have a large family?
B: Yes, I have a large family.
A: Who are the members of your family?

B: I have two sons and three daughters.
A: Are there any others who live with you?
B: Yes, my wife's grandmother lives with us.

A: ¿Qué tal su familia?
B: Mis padres tienen muchos problemas.
A: ¿Qué problemas tienen?
A: Mi padre no tiene trabajo.
B: ¿Tiene trabajo su madre?
A: Sí, pero no gana mucho dinero.

A: How is your family?
B: My parents have a lot of problems.
A: What problems do they have?
B: My father doesn't have a job.
A: Does your mother have a job?
B: Yes, but she doesn't make much money.

A: ¿En qué trabaja Ud.?
B: Soy hombre de negocios.

A: What work do you do?
B: I'm a businessman.

A: ¿En qué trabaja su mujer?

B: Es secretaria en una compañía de seguros.

A: ¿Tiene Ud. hijos?

B: Sí, tengo dos hijos. El menor trabaja conmigo. El mayor es actor.

A: What does your wife do?

B: She's a secretary in an insurance company.

A: Do you have children?

B: Yes, I have two sons. The younger one works with me. The older one is an actor.

Vocabulary

CARDINAL NUMBERS

0	~~zero~~ *cero*	27	veinte y siete, veintisiete
*1	uno, un, una	28	veinte y ocho, veintiocho
2	dos	29	veinte y nueve, veintinueve
3	tres	30	treinta
4	cuatro	31	treinta y uno, un, una
5	cinco	32	treinta y dos
6	seis	40	cuarenta
7	siete	50	cincuenta
8	ocho	60	sesenta
9	nueve	70	setenta
10	diez	80	ochenta
11	once	90	noventa — *used ā another number*
12	doce	*100	ciento, cien - *used ā a noun*
13	trece	101	ciento uno
14	catorce	102	ciento dos
15	quince	200	doscientos,-as
*16	diez y seis, dieciséis	300	trescientos,-as
17	diez y siete, diecisiete	400	cuatrocientos,-as
18	diez y ocho, dieciocho	*500	quinientos,-as
19	diez y nueve, diecinueve	600	seiscientos,-as
20	veinte	*700	setecientos,-as
21	veinte y uno, veinte y un, veinte y una; veintiuno, veintiún, veintiuna	800	ochocientos,-as
		*900	novecientos,-as
22	veinte y dos, veintidós	1,000	mil
23	veinte y tres, veintitrés	2,000	dos mil
24	veinte y cuatro, veinticuatro	*100,000	cien mil
25	veinte y cinco, veinticinco	1,000,000	un millón
26	veinte y seis, veintiséis	2,000,000	dos millones

* **Uno** becomes **un** before masculine nouns (**un libro**) and **una** before feminine nouns (**una casa, veinte y una casas**). The numerals from two hundred (**doscientos**) to nine hundred (**novecientos**) have feminine plural forms (**doscientas, trescientas,** etc.). Numbers sixteen (**diez y seis**) to nineteen (**diez y nueve**) may be written as one word (**dieciséis,** etc.); also the numbers twenty-one to twenty-nine. Note that the numbers sixteen (**dieciséis**), twenty-two (**veintidós**), twenty-three (**veintitrés**), and twenty-six (**veintiséis**) carry an accent on the last syllable. The conjunction **y** (*and*) appears in numbers sixteen to ninety-nine. **Ciento** becomes **cien** before nouns and before the words **mil** and **millones.** Note the spelling of **quinientos, setecientos,** and **novecientos.**

ORDINAL NUMBERS

*primero,-a	*first*	sexto,-a	*sixth*
segundo,-a	*second*	séptimo,-a	*seventh*
*tercero,-a	*third*	octavo,-a	*eighth*
cuarto,-a	*fourth*	noveno,-a	*ninth*
quinto,-a	*fifth*	décimo,-a	*tenth*

Grammar

HOW AGE IS EXPRESSED

The Spanish equivalent of the expression *How old are you?* is **¿Cuántos años tiene Ud.?** (literally, *How many years do you have?*).

¿Cuántos años tiene él? *How old is he?*
Él tiene catorce años. *He's fourteen years old.*

Oral practice

1. ¿Cuántos años tiene el médico? • 42
2. ¿Cuántos años tiene su madre? • 65
3. ¿Cuántos años tiene Ud.? • 35
4. ¿Cuántos años tiene el paciente? • 22
5. ¿Cuántos años tiene su marido? • 33
6. ¿Cuántos años tiene su hija? • 12
7. ¿Cuántos años tiene su abuelo? • 89
8. ¿Cuántos años tiene su abuela? • 77
9. ¿Cuántos años tiene el señor Pérez? • 43
10. ¿Cuántos años tiene la enfermera? • 27

Grammar

TELLING TIME

Telling time in Spanish is fairly similar to telling time in English. The verb **ser** is used with the appropriate definite article and the number or numbers. In the case of one o'clock, the singular forms of the verb and article are used.

Es la una. *It's one o'clock.*

For all other hours, the plural forms of the verb and article are used.

Son las dos. *It's two o'clock.*

---

* The forms **primero** and **tercero** drop the final **-o** when they precede masculine singular nouns (**el primer libro, el tercer hospital**). Beyond tenth (**décimo,-a**) cardinal numbers are used.

®️ *side of clock*

To express time after the hour, add **y.** To express time before the hour, add **menos** (*less*).

Son las dos y diez.	*It's ten past two.*
Son las tres menos diez.	*It's ten to three.*

For the half hour, use the word **media;** for the quarter hour, **cuarto.**

Ⓛ *side of clock*

Son las cuatro y media.	*It's half past four.*
Son las cinco y cuarto.	*It's quarter past five.*
Son las seis menos cuarto.	*It's a quarter to six.*

Asking the time is also very similar to English, the principal difference being that the word **hour** is substituted for the word **time.** The singular form of the verb is always used in asking what time (which hour) it is.

¿Qué hora es?	*What time is it?*
¿A qué hora es la clase?	*At what time is the class?*
¿A qué hora llega el autobús?	*At what time does the bus come?*

Instead of A.M. and P.M., Spanish uses the following expressions for parts of the day and night:

de la madrugada *midnight to dawn*	**de la noche** *dusk to midnight*
de la mañana *dawn to noon*	**la medianoche** *midnight*
de la tarde *noon to dusk*	**el mediodía** *noon*

Oral practice

Answer the questions by following the model.

¿Qué hora es? ¿Son las dos?	*What time is it? Is it two o'clock?*
No, son las dos y cuarto.	*No, it's a quarter past two.*

1. ¿Qué hora es? ¿Son las tres?
2. ¿Qué hora es? ¿Son las cuatro?
3. ¿Qué hora es? ¿Son las cinco?
4. ¿Qué hora es? ¿Son las seis?
5. ¿Qué hora es? ¿Son las siete?
6. ¿Qué hora es? ¿Son las ocho?
7. ¿Qué hora es? ¿Son las nueve?

¿A qué hora es la cita? A la una?	*At what time is the appointment? At one?*
No, es a la una y media.	*No, it's at one thirty.*

1. ¿A qué hora es la cita? ¿A las cinco?
2. ¿A qué hora es la cita? ¿A las seis?
3. ¿A qué hora es la cita? ¿A las siete?
4. ¿A qué hora es la cita? ¿A las ocho?
5. ¿A qué hora es la cita? ¿A las nueve?
6. ¿A qué hora es la cita? ¿A las diez?
7. ¿A qué hora es la cita? ¿A las once?

¿Cuándo llega el médico? ¿A las nueve?

No, él llega a las diez menos cuarto.

When does the doctor arrive? At nine?

No, he arrives at quarter to ten.

1. ¿Cuándo llega el médico? ¿A las doce?
2. ¿Cuándo llega el médico? ¿A las cinco?
3. ¿Cuándo llega el médico? ¿A las tres?
4. ¿Cuándo llega el médico? ¿A la una?
5. ¿Cuándo llega el médico? ¿A las diez?
6. ¿Cuándo llega el médico? ¿A las dos y cuarto?
7. ¿Cuándo llega el médico? ¿A las cuatro y media?

Written practice

Write out these times in Spanish.

1. 3:47 A.M.	8. 7:30 P.M.	15. 6:45 P.M.
2. 5:13 P.M.	9. 12:30 P.M.	16. 7:55 A.M.
3. 6:27 A.M.	10. 9:45 A.M.	17. 1:25 A.M.
4. 10:22 P.M.	11. 1:10 P.M.	18. 9:12 P.M.
5. 12:00 noon	12. 8:16 A.M.	19. 5:47 A.M.
6. 11:35 A.M.	13. 2:25 P.M.	20. 12:00 midnight
7. 4:50 A.M.	14. 10:50 A.M.	

Vocabulary

THE DAYS OF THE WEEK/LOS DÍAS DE LA SEMANA

lunes *Monday*

martes *Tuesday*

miércoles *Wednesday*

jueves *Thursday*

viernes *Friday*

sábado *Saturday*

domingo *Sunday*

Other words and expressions commonly used in speaking of the time or day include:

hoy *today*

mañana *tomorrow*

ayer *yesterday*

anteayer *day before yesterday*

pasado mañana *day after tomorrow*

¿Qué día es hoy? *What day is today?*

Oral practice

Answer the questions using the cues.

¿Cuándo es la cita?

La cita es el lunes a las tres y media.

When is the appointment?

The appointment is Monday at 3:30.

1. ¿Cuándo es la cita?
   • Tuesday at 4:15   • Thursday at 6:20   • Wednesday at 7:30

2. ¿A qué hora llega la doctora?
   ● Friday at 7:30   ● Saturday at 12:45   ● Monday at 2:50

3. ¿Cuándo tenemos que regresar?
   ● Sunday at 1:00   ● Wednesday at 8:10   ● Tuesday at 11:30

Conversations

A: ¿Cuándo es su cita con el especialista?

A: When is your appointment with the specialist?

B: Es el lunes a las cuatro de la tarde pero tengo que cambiar el día.

B: It's on Monday at four in the afternoon but I have to change the day.

A: ¿Por qué?

A: Why?

B: Porque los lunes trabajo hasta las cuatro y media.

B: Because on Mondays I work until four-thirty.

A: ¿Es conveniente el martes a las cinco?

A: Is Tuesday at five convenient?

B: Sí, muchas gracias.

B: Yes, thank you very much.

A: ¿Cuál es su dirección?

A: What is your address?

B: Vivo en el número treinta de la calle cuarenta y tres.

B: I live at 30 Forty-third Street.

A: ¿Es una casa particular o un apartamento?

A: Is it a private house or an apartment?

B: Es un apartamento, número 3C.

B: It's an apartment, number 3C.

A: ¿Cuál es su número de teléfono?

A: What is your telephone number?

B: Mi número de teléfono es 372-4986.

B: My telephone number is 372-4986.

A: ¿Cuál es su dirección?

A: What is your address?

B: Vivo en el número setenta y dos de la calle diez.

B: I live at 72 Tenth Street.

A: ¿Cuál es su número de teléfono?

A: What is your telephone number?

B: Mi número de teléfono es 654-4781.

B: My telephone number is 654-4781.

A: ¿Cuál es su número de seguro social?

A: What is your Social Security number?

B: Mi número de seguro social es 462-33-0817.

B: My Social Security number is 462-33-0817.

Dialogue

RECEPCIONISTA: El hospital necesita alguna información de Ud. en caso de emergencia.
PACIENTE: Comprendo. (Entiendo.)
RECEPCIONISTA: Primero, ¿cuántos años tiene Ud.? (¿Qué edad?)
PACIENTE: Tengo treinta y cuatro años.
RECEPCIONISTA: ¿De dónde es Ud.?
PACIENTE: Soy de Puerto Rico.
RECEPCIONISTA: ¿En qué trabaja Ud.?

PACIENTE: Soy carpintero.
RECEPCIONISTA: ¿Es Ud. casado?
PACIENTE: Sí, soy casado.
RECEPCIONISTA: ¿Trabaja su esposa?
PACIENTE: Sí, ella trabaja en una fábrica.
RECEPCIONISTA: ¿Tiene Ud. hijos?
PACIENTE: Sí, tengo tres; un hijo y dos hijas.
RECEPCIONISTA: ¿Cuántos años tienen ellos?
PACIENTE: El muchacho tiene nueve años y las dos muchachas tienen siete y once años.
RECEPCIONISTA: *¿A quién avisamos en caso de emergencia?
PACIENTE: *Tienen que avisar a mis padres porque mi mujer trabaja. Su número de teléfono es 231-6247.
RECEPCIONISTA: Muy bien. Ahora Ud. tiene que llenar el formulario y firmar aquí.

VOCABULARY

alguno(-a) *some*
en caso de emergencia *in case of emergency*
primero *first*
casado(-a) *married*
con *with*
la fábrica *factory*

el muchacho *boy*
la muchacha *girl*
avisar *to notify*
llenar *to fill out, to fill a Rx, to fill a container c liquid*
el formulario *form, application*
firmar *to sign*
aquí *here*

RECEPTIONIST: The hospital needs some information from you in case of emergency.
PATIENT: I understand.
RECEPTIONIST: First, how old are you?
PATIENT: I'm thirty-four years old.
RECEPTIONIST: Where are you from?
PATIENT: I'm from Puerto Rico.
RECEPTIONIST: What work do you do?
PATIENT: I'm a carpenter.
RECEPTIONIST: Are you married?
PATIENT: Yes, I'm married.
RECEPTIONIST: Does your wife work?
PATIENT: Yes, she works in a factory.
RECEPTIONIST: Do you have any children?
PATIENT: Yes, I have three; a son and two daughters.
RECEPTIONIST: How old are they?
PATIENT: The boy is nine years old and the two girls are seven and eleven years old.
RECEPTIONIST: Whom do we notify in case of emergency?

* Whenever a person is the direct object of the verb, the direct object must be preceded by the preposition **a.** This is called the personal **a.**

PATIENT: You have to notify my parents because my wife works. Their telephone
                number is 231-6247.
RECEPTIONIST: Very well. Now you must fill out the form and sign here.

QUESTIONS ON DIALOGUE

1. ¿Qué necesita el hospital?
2. ¿Cuántos años tiene el paciente?
3. ¿De dónde es el paciente?
4. ¿En qué trabaja el paciente?
5. ¿Es casado el paciente?
6. ¿Trabaja su esposa? ¿Dónde trabaja?
7. ¿Tiene hijos el paciente?
8. ¿Cuántos años tienen sus hijos?
9. ¿A quién notifica el hospital en caso de emergencia?
10. ¿Qué tiene que hacer el paciente?

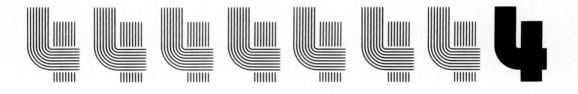

Grammar

PRESENT INDICATIVE OF THE IRREGULAR VERB *ESTAR* (TO BE)

yo	**estoy**	*I am*
él/ella	**está**	*he/she is*
usted (Ud.)	**está**	*you are*
nosotros/nosotras	**estamos**	*we are*
ellos/ellas	**están**	*they are*
ustedes (Uds.)	**están**	*you* (pl.) *are*

The verb **estar** also means *to be,* but it is used to refer to a state or condition—as, for example, the state of a person's health.

¿Cómo está Ud. hoy?	*How are you today?*
Estoy bien, gracias.	*I'm well, thank you.*
¿Cómo está el paciente?	*How is the patient?*
El paciente está mal.	*The patient is ill.*

The verb **estar** is also used to indicate the position or location of a person, place, or thing. For example:

¿Dónde está el médico?	*Where is the doctor?*
El médico está en la cafetería.	*The doctor is in the cafeteria.*
¿Dónde está la clínica?	*Where is the clinic?*
La clínica está en la ciudad.	*The clinic is in the city.*
¿Dónde está la receta?	*Where is the prescription?*
La receta está en la farmacia.	*The prescription is in the pharmacy.*

Oral practice

Answer the questions by following the model.

¿Cómo están los pacientes?   *How are the patients?*
Los pacientes están bien.   *The patients are well.*

1. ¿Cómo está el médico?
2. ¿Cómo están las enfermeras?
3. ¿Cómo está la paciente?
4. ¿Cómo están los muchachos?
5. ¿Cómo están las muchachas?
6. ¿Cómo está el hombre?
7. ¿Cómo están las mujeres?
8. ¿Cómo está la madre?
9. ¿Cómo están los padres?
10. ¿Cómo está la muchacha?

Answer the questions by following the model.

¿Cómo están sus padres?   *How are your parents?*
Mis padres están mal.   *My parents are ill.*

1. ¿Cómo está su madre?
2. ¿Cómo están sus tíos?
3. ¿Cómo está su suegra?
4. ¿Cómo están sus hermanos?
5. ¿Cómo está su marido?
6. ¿Cómo están sus primos?
7. ¿Cómo está su esposa?
8. ¿Cómo está su suegro?
9. ¿Cómo están sus sobrinos?
10. ¿Cómo están sus hijos?

Answer the questions using the cues.

¿Dónde está el médico?   *Where is the doctor?*
El médico está en la clínica.   *The doctor is in the clinic.*

1. ¿Dónde está la paciente?   • room
2. ¿Dónde está el técnico?   • laboratory
3. ¿Dónde está el farmacéutico?   • pharmacy
4. ¿Dónde están los hombres?   • cities
5. ¿Dónde están las enfermeras?   • hospitals
6. ¿Dónde está la madre?   • factory
7. ¿Dónde está la mujer?   • cafeteria
8. ¿Dónde está el hombre?   • house
9. ¿Dónde está el muchacho?   • living room
10. ¿Dónde está la psiquiatra?   • office

Change the sentences to the plural by following the model.

El médico está en la sala de emergencia.	*The doctor is in the emergency room.*
Los médicos están en las salas de emergencia.	*The doctors are in the emergency rooms.*

1. El hombre está en el hospital.
2. La enfermera está en la ciudad.
3. El óptico está en la oficina.
4. La pediatra está en la clínica.
5. El técnico está en el laboratorio.
6. El policía está en la casa.
7. La psicóloga está en la cafetería.
8. El farmacéutico está en la farmacia.
9. La madre está en la sala de emergencia.
10. El muchacho está en el cuarto.

Grammar

ADJECTIVES

Adjectives that indicate a state or condition are used with the verb **estar.** For example:

El paciente está preocupado.	*The patient is worried.*
La muchacha está nerviosa.	*The girl is nervous.*
Las mujeres están ocupadas.	*The women are busy.*
Yo estoy cansado.	*I am tired.*

Some adjectives have different meanings when they are used with either **ser** or **estar.**

Él es listo.	*He is clever.*
Él está listo.	*He is ready.*
Mi tío es aburrido.	*My uncle is boring.*
Mi tío está aburrido.	*My uncle is bored.*
Él es borracho.	*He is a drunkard.*
Él está borracho.	*He is drunk.*

Certain other adjectives, although they will not change meaning, will have a different implication depending upon their use with either **ser** or **estar.**

Ella es pálida.	*She is pale (a pale girl).*
Ella está pálida hoy.	*She is pale today (a condition).*
José es alegre.	*José is happy (a happy person).*
José está alegre hoy.	*José is happy (in a happy mood).*
Carmen es bonita.	*Carmen is pretty (a pretty girl).*
Carmen está bonita hoy.	*Carmen is pretty (looks pretty).*

Oral practice

Change the following to the plural. Make sure that the adjectives agree in gender and number with the nouns that they describe.

1. El cuarto está vacío (*empty*).
2. La botella está llena (*full*).
3. El libro está cerrado (*closed*).
4. La farmacia está abierta (*open*).
5. El vaso está limpio (*clean*).
6. La taza está sucia (*dirty*).
7. El hombre está sentado (*seated*).
8. La mujer está parada (*standing*).
9. El paciente está dormido (*asleep*).
10. La paciente está despierta (*awake*).
11. El muchacho está tranquilo (*calm*).
12. La muchacha está agitada (*upset*).
13. El anciano está triste (*sad*).
14. La anciana está alegre (*happy*).

Answer the following questions.

1. ¿Está molesto (*uncomfortable*) el muchacho?
2. ¿Está aturdida (*giddy*) la joven?
3. ¿Está enferma (*ill*) la madre?
4. ¿Están enojados (*angry*) Uds.?
5. ¿Está fría (*cold*) la cerveza?
6. ¿Están confusas (*confused*) las jóvenes?
7. ¿Están inquietos (*restless*) los pacientes?
8. ¿Está sobrio (*sober*) el hombre?
9. ¿Está caliente (*hot*) el café?
10. ¿Está contenta (*happy*) la madre?

Conversations

A: ¿Por qué está Ud. en la ciudad?
B: Tengo que consultar con un psiquiatra.
A: ¿Por qué? ¿Cuál es su problema?
B: No estoy bien. Sufro de los nervios.

A: ¿Está su mujer en la ciudad también?
B: No. Ella está en casa con nuestros hijos.

A: Why are you in the city?
B: I have to consult with a psychiatrist.
A: Why? What is your problem?
B: I'm not well. I'm suffering from nervousness.

A: Is your wife in the city also?
B: No. She's at home with our children.

A: ¿Cómo está Ud.?
B: Estoy muy bien, gracias.
A: Y sus padres, ¿cómo están ellos?
B: Mi padre no está bien.
A: ¿Por qué? ¿Qué tiene?
B: Está muy débil y no tiene apetito.

A: How are you?
B: I'm fine, thanks.
A: And your parents, how are they?
B: My father isn't well.
A: Why? What's wrong with him?
B: He's very weak and he doesn't have an appetite.

A: ¿Cómo está el paciente en el cuarto nueve?
B: No está bien.
A: ¿Por qué? ¿Qué tiene?
B: Tiene pulmonía.
A: ¿Está muy mal?
B: Sí, está muy mal porque es anciano.

A: How is the patient in room nine?
B: He's not well.
A: Why? What's wrong with him?
B: He has pneumonia.
A: Is he seriously ill?
B: Yes, he's very ill because he's a very old person.

Written practice

Translate the sentences into Spanish.

1. The patient (*masc.*) is very restless and doesn't have an appetite.
2. How is the patient (*fem.*) in room fifty-seven?
3. Where is my doctor?
4. The woman is worried because her son is in the hospital.
5. The technician is in the laboratory.
6. We have to be in the hospital at nine A.M.
7. My wife is not in the city.
8. Where are your children?
9. The doctor is very busy today.
10. My husband is in the living room.

Grammar

REFLEXIVE PRONOUNS AND VERBS

The reflexive pronouns are:

me   *myself*
nos   *ourselves*
se   *himself, herself, yourself, themselves, yourselves*

Reflexive pronouns are used to indicate that the subject of the sentence is the person acted upon by the verb. Some reflexive verbs are:

bañar<u>se</u>   *to bathe oneself*
cansar<u>se</u>   *to tire oneself*

lavar<u>se</u>   *to wash oneself*
levantar<u>se</u>   *to stand up, to get up*

The reflexive pronoun usually precedes the verb in a sentence.

El hombre se baña.	*The man is bathing himself.*
Me canso fácilmente.	*I tire easily.*

If a reflexive verb is used non-reflexively, it will have a different meaning. For example:

El paciente se baña.	*The patient is bathing himself.*
La enfermera baña al paciente.	*The nurse is bathing the patient.*

Some verbs are reflexive in Spanish even though the reflexive meaning may not be apparent in English. Such verbs must be learned as reflexive verbs.

Oral practice

Change the sentences using the cues.

El muchacho se baña.	*The boy is bathing himself.*
Nosotras nos bañamos.	*We are bathing ourselves.*

1. Las mujeres se cansan.
   • yo   • el paciente   • el médico   • las enfermeras

2. Mi padre se lava todos los días.
   • nosotros   • mis padres   • mi hijo   • la paciente

3. El hombre se levanta a las siete de la mañana.
   • el técnico   • el especialista   • la recepcionista   • las pacientes

Grammar

PRESENT INDICATIVE OF THE REFLEXIVE VERB *LLAMARSE** (TO BE CALLED)

yo	**me llamo**	*my name is*
él/ella	**se llama**	*his/her name is*
Ud.	**se llama**	*your name is*

nosotros/nosotras	**nos llamamos**	*our names are*
ellos/ellas	**se llaman**	*their names are*
Uds.	**se llaman**	*your (pl.) names are*

Llamarse literally means *to call oneself,* but it is the normal way of saying what one's name is. To ask a person's name, one uses the interrogative **¿cómo?** with the verb **llamarse.**

¿Cómo se llama Ud.?	*What is your name?*
Me llamo Juan López.	*My name is Juan López.*

* The infinitive form of reflexive verbs is written with the third person singular pronoun attached to the end of the verb, hence **llamar + se = llamarse.**

¿Cómo se llama el enfermo?
Se llama Héctor Rivera.

What is the sick man's name?
His name is Héctor Rivera.

¿Cómo se llama la enferma?
Se llama Ana Martínez.

What is the sick woman's name?
Her name is Ana Martínez.

¿Cómo se llama el hospital?
Se llama General Hospital.

What is the hospital called?
It's called General Hospital.

Oral practice

Answer the questions with complete sentences. If necessary, use your imagination.

1. ¿Cómo se llama Ud.?
2. ¿Cómo se llama su esposo?
3. ¿Cómo se llama su esposa?
4. ¿Cómo se llama su madre?
5. ¿Cómo se llama su padre?
6. ¿Cómo se llama su hija?
7. ¿Cómo se llama su hijo?
8. ¿Cómo se llaman sus hermanas?
9. ¿Cómo se llaman sus hermanos?
10. ¿Cómo se llama su médico?

Conversations

A: ¿Cómo se llama Ud.?
B: Me llamo Inés Rodríguez.
A: ¿Cómo se llama su esposo?
B: Se llama Jorge.
A: ¿Viven Uds. en una casa privada o en un apartamento?
B: Vivimos en un apartamento.

A: What is your name?
B: My name is Inés Rodríguez.
A: What is your husband's name?
B: His name is Jorge.
A: Do you live in a private house or in an apartment?
B: We live in an apartment.

A: ¿A qué hora se levanta Ud. por la mañana?
B: Me levanto a las seis y media, y me baño.
A: ¿A qué hora toma Ud. el desayuno?
B: Tomo el desayuno a las siete y cuarto.
A: ¿En qué trabaja Ud.?
B: Soy mecánico.

A: What time do you get up in the morning?
B: I get up at six-thirty and I bathe.
A: What time do you have breakfast?
B: I have breakfast at seven-fifteen.
A: What work do you do?
B: I am a mechanic.

A: Señor, Ud. tiene que levantarse ahora.
B: ¿Por qué tengo que levantarme?
A: Porque tiene que bañarse.
B: Pero es muy temprano todavía.

A: Sir, you must get up now.
B: Why must I get up?
A: Because you have to bathe yourself.
B: But it is still very early.

A: No, no es temprano, es muy tarde.
B: ¿Qué hora es?
A: Son las once y media de la mañana.

A: No, it is not early, it is very late.
B: What time is it?
A: It is eleven-thirty A.M.

VOCABULARY

el aire acondicionado air conditioning
la almohada pillow
el asistente orderly, aide
la asistenta aide
la autorización authorization, consent
la calefacción heating
la cama bed
el catéter catheter
la cirugía surgery
el colchón mattress
el enfermero male nurse
la enfermera female nurse
la enfermera auxiliar nurse's aide

el examen médico medical examination
las horas de visita visiting hours
la inyección injection
la inyección intravenosa intravenous injection
la manta blanket
la operación operation
los puntos stitches
la prueba test
el reconocimiento médico medical examination
las reglas rules
el ruido noise
las sábanas sheets

Oral practice

Answer the questions using the cues.

¿De qué se queja el hijo?
El hijo se queja de la comida.

What is the son complaining about?
The son is complaining about the food.

1. ¿De qué se queja el enfermo?
2. ¿De qué se queja la enferma?
3. ¿De qué se queja la mujer?
4. ¿De qué se queja el hombre?
5. ¿De qué se quejan los pacientes?
6. ¿De qué se queja la muchacha?
7. ¿De qué se queja la madre?
8. ¿De qué se queja el padre?
9. ¿De qué se queja el anciano?
10. ¿De qué se queja el muchacho?

- pillow
- bed
- catheter
- operation
- heating
- stitches
- noise
- visiting hours
- tests
- rules

Grammar

PRESENT INDICATIVE OF THE IRREGULAR VERB *DESPERTARSE* (TO WAKE UP)

yo	**me despierto**	*I wake up*
él/ella	**se despierta**	*he/she wakes up*
Ud.	**se despierta**	*you wake up*

nosotros/nosotras	**nos despertamos**	*we wake up*
ellos/ellas	**se despiertan**	*they wake up*
Uds.	**se despiertan**	*you* (pl.) *wake up*

When used reflexively, this verb means *to wake up.* When it is used non-reflexively, it means *to wake someone up.* For example:

| **La muchacha se despierta a las seis.** | *The girl wakes up at six.* |
| **Ella despierta al paciente a las siete.** | *She wakes the patient at seven.* |

Oral practice

Change the sentences using the cues.

1. La madre se despierta temprano todos los días.
   - el hombre   • las enfermeras   • los pacientes   • yo

2. El muchacho se despierta tarde (*late*) todos los días.
   - los muchachos   • las mujeres   • nosotros   • la muchacha

Grammar

PRESENT INDICATIVE OF THE IRREGULAR VERB *ACOSTARSE* (TO GO TO BED)

yo	**me acuesto**	*I go to bed*
él/ella	**se acuesta**	*he/she goes to bed*
Ud.	**se acuesta**	*you go to bed*
nosotros/nosotras	**nos acostamos**	*we go to bed*
ellos/ellas	**se acuestan**	*they go to bed*
Uds.	**se acuestan**	*you* (pl.) *go to bed*

This verb when used reflexively means *to go to bed.* It can also be used non-reflexively meaning *to put someone to bed.*

Oral practice

Change the sentences using the cues.

1. La enfermera se acuesta tarde cada noche.
   - el especialista   • la asistenta   • la enfermera auxiliar   • el enfermero

2. La muchacha se acuesta temprano cada noche.
   - la mujer   • el muchacho   • nosotros   • los muchachos

Answer the questions with complete sentences.

1. ¿A qué hora se despierta Ud. por la mañana?
2. ¿A qué hora se acuesta Ud. por la noche?

3. ¿Se despierta Ud. temprano todas las mañanas?
4. ¿Se acuesta Ud. tarde cada noche?
5. ¿A qué hora despierta el padre a sus hijos?
6. ¿A qué hora acuesta la madre a sus hijos?
7. ¿A qué hora tienen que despertarse los pacientes?
8. ¿A qué hora tienen que acostarse los pacientes?
9. ¿A qué hora tienen que despertarse sus hijos?
10. ¿A qué hora tienen que acostarse sus hijos?

Written practice

Translate the sentences into Spanish.

1. The technician is in the laboratory.
2. The man is drunk.
3. I must get up early tomorrow.
4. Why do I tire easily?
5. The woman is complaining about the noise.
6. What is the sick woman's name?
7. Where are you from?
8. How is your wife?
9. What time do you get up in the morning?

Grammar

DEMONSTRATIVE ADJECTIVES AND PRONOUNS

| | ADJECTIVES | | PRONOUNS | | |
	masculine	feminine	masculine	feminine	neuter
this	este	esta	éste	ésta	esto
that	ese	esa	ése	ésa	eso
these	estos	estas	éstos	éstas	
those	esos	esas	ésos	ésas	

Demonstrative adjectives precede the nouns they modify. They must agree with these nouns in gender and number. For example:

Leo este periódico.   *I'm reading this newspaper.*
Necesitamos esas revistas.   *We need those magazines.*

Demonstrative pronouns are identical to the demonstrative adjectives except that they carry an accent mark. They are used to refer to a noun that is not present, and the singular forms are often translated *this one* and *that one.*

Leo éste.   *I'm reading this one.*
Necesitamos ésas.   *We need those.*

The neuter forms of the demonstrative pronouns do not carry accent marks. The neuter forms are used to refer to ideas or situations rather than to specific nouns. For example:

No creo esto.	*I don't believe this.*
No comprendo eso.	*I don't understand that.*

Oral practice

Repeat the sentences after your instructor.

El paciente toma esta píldora.	El paciente toma este periódico.
El paciente toma ésta.	El paciente toma éste.
El paciente toma estas píldoras.	El paciente toma estos periódicos.
El paciente toma éstas.	El paciente toma éstos.
El paciente toma esa píldora.	El paciente toma ese periódico.
El paciente toma ésa.	El paciente toma ése.
El paciente toma esas píldoras.	El paciente toma esos periódicos.
El paciente toma ésas.	El paciente toma ésos.

Written practice

Translate the words in italics into Spanish.

1. Necesito *these* píldoras.
2. *This* médico es muy agradable.
3. *These* pacientes están muy graves.
4. *These* enfermeras son muy competentes.
5. Necesito leer *that* revista.
6. *This* medicina es buena.
7. *Those* ventanas están limpias.
8. Tengo que comprar *those* píldoras.
9. El médico analiza *these* problemas.
10. Tenemos que abrir *this* puerta.

Dialogue

ENFERMERA: ¿Cómo está Ud. hoy, señora Moreno?
PACIENTE: No estoy bien. Estoy inquieta y nerviosa. Tengo miedo.
ENFERMERA: No debe tener miedo, señora.
PACIENTE: Mi familia no está aquí. Tengo miedo de la operación mañana.
ENFERMERA: ¿Dónde está su familia?

PACIENTE: Mi familia está en casa.

ENFERMERA: Ud. debe calmarse. No hay problema. Es una operación sencilla. ¿Está Ud. cansada?

PACIENTE: Sí, estoy muy cansada.

ENFERMERA: Ud. debe estar tranquila. ¿Por qué no toma Ud. un calmante con un vaso de agua?

PACIENTE: Muchas gracias, señorita. Ud. es muy amable. Ahora estoy tranquila.

VOCABULARY

deber (+ infinitive) *must, ought to, should*

aquí *here*

en casa *at home*

calmarse *to calm down*

hay *there is, there are*

sencillo(-a) *simple*

el calmante *sedative*

el vaso *glass*

NURSE: How are you today, Mrs. Moreno?

PATIENT: I'm not well. I'm restless and nervous. I'm frightened.

NURSE: You should not be frightened, ma'am.

PATIENT: My family isn't here. I'm afraid of tomorrow's operation.

NURSE: Where is your family?

PATIENT: My family is at home.

NURSE: You must calm down. There's no problem. It's a simple operation. Are you tired?

PATIENT: Yes, I'm very tired.

NURSE: You should be calm. Why don't you take a sedative with a glass of water?

PATIENT: Thank you very much, miss. You are very kind. I'm calm now.

QUESTIONS ON DIALOGUE

1. ¿Cómo está la señora Moreno?
2. ¿Dónde está su familia?
3. ¿De qué se queja?
4. ¿De qué tiene miedo?
5. ¿Qué toma para calmarse?

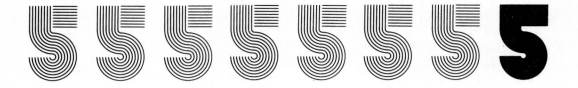

Vocabulary

PARTS OF THE BODY: THE HEAD/PARTES DEL CUERPO: LA CABEZA

el cuero cabelludo *scalp*
el pelo *hair*
el cabello *hair*
la frente *forehead*
la sien *temple*
las cejas *eyebrows*
los párpados *eyelids*
las pestañas *eyelashes*
el ojo *eye*
el globo del ojo *eyeball*
la pupila *pupil*
la oreja *outer ear, earlobe*
el oído *inner ear, hearing*
la nariz *nose*
las fosas nasales *nostrils*
las mejillas *cheeks*

los cachetes *cheeks*
la boca *mouth*
los labios *lips*
los dientes *teeth*
las muelas *teeth*
las encías *gums*
la lengua *tongue*
las amígdalas *tonsils*
la garganta *throat*
la barbilla *chin*
el mentón *chin*
la quijada *jaw*
la mandíbula *jaw*
el cuello *neck*
la nuez de Adán *Adam's apple*
la nuca *nape of neck*

Oral practice

Answer the questions with complete sentences.

1. ¿Tiene Ud. dolor de cabeza?
*2. ¿Tienen Uds. dolor en los ojos?
3. ¿Tiene la paciente dolor en el ojo derecho (*right eye*)?
4. ¿Tiene el hombre dolor en el ojo izquierdo (*left eye*)?

In Spanish, the definite article is generally used instead of the possessive adjective when referring to parts of the body.

5. ¿Tiene el paciente dolor de los oídos?
6. ¿Tiene Ud. dolor del oído derecho?
7. ¿Tiene Ud. dolor del oído izquierdo?
8. ¿Tiene la mujer dolor en la frente?
9. ¿Tiene la muchacha dolor en la boca?
10. ¿Tiene el muchacho dolor de muelas?

Answer the questions with original responses. Use complete sentences.

1. ¿Dónde tiene Ud. dolor?
2. ¿Dónde tiene dolor el enfermo?
3. ¿Dónde tiene dolor su esposa?
4. ¿Dónde tiene dolor su esposo?
5. ¿Dónde tiene dolor su madre?
6. ¿Dónde tiene dolor su padre?
7. ¿Dónde tienen dolor los pacientes?
8. ¿Dónde tiene dolor su hermana?
9. ¿Dónde tiene dolor su hijo?
10. ¿Dónde tiene dolor su abuelo?

Grammar

PRESENT INDICATIVE OF THE IRREGULAR VERB *SENTIRSE* (TO FEEL)

yo	**me siento**	*I feel*
él/ella	**se siente**	*he/she feels*
Ud.	**se siente**	*you feel*
nosotros/nosotras	**nos sentimos**	*we feel*
ellos/ellas	**se sienten**	*they feel*
Uds.	**se sienten**	*you* (pl.) *feel*

Oral practice

Change the sentences using the cues.

1. Los pacientes se sienten bien.
   • yo   • mi hermano y yo   • mi marido   • mis tíos

2. El hombre se siente mal.
   • mis padres   • los muchachos   • mis padres y yo   • mi hermana

Change to the plural.

1. Me siento mal.
2. La paciente se siente mal.
3. Mi hermano se siente mal.
4. El policía se siente mal.
5. El hombre de negocios se siente mal.

Change to the singular.

1. Nos sentimos mal.
2. Mis primos se sienten mal.
3. Las secretarias se sienten mal.
4. Las enfermeras se sienten mal.
5. Los técnicos se sienten mal.

Change the sentences using the cues.

1. La mujer se siente nerviosa.
2. El paciente se siente cansado.
3. El enfermero se siente agitado.
4. El padre se siente confuso.
5. El muchacho se siente aturdido.

- los hombres
- las pacientes
- las enfermeras
- la madre
- la muchacha

Answer the questions with complete sentences.

1. ¿Siente Ud. dolor en la frente?
2. ¿Siente Ud. dolor en la nariz?
3. ¿Siente Ud. dolor de cabeza?
4. ¿Siente Ud. dolor de muelas?
5. ¿Siente Ud. dolor del oído?

Conversations

A: ¿Cómo se siente Ud. hoy?
B: No muy bien.
A: ¿Por qué? ¿Qué tiene?
B: Siento irritación en el ojo izquierdo.
A: ¿Qué toma Ud. para la irritación?
B: Tomo estas gotas.

A: How are you feeling today?
B: Not very well.
A: Why? What's wrong?
B: My left eye feels irritated.
A: What are you taking for the irritation?
B: I'm taking these drops.

A: ¿Cómo están sus padres?
B: Mi padre está bien pero mi madre no.
A: ¿Qué tiene ella?
B: Tiene dolor de muelas.
A: ¿Por qué no visita al dentista?
B: Porque tiene miedo.

A: How are your parents?
B: My father is well but my mother isn't.
A: What's wrong with her?
B: She has a toothache.
A: Why doesn't she visit the dentist?
B: Because she's frightened.

A: ¿Cómo se siente su marido?
B: No está bien.
A: ¿Cuál es su problema?
B: Sufre de dolores del oído.
A: ¿Por qué no consultan Uds. con un especialista?
B: Porque no tenemos bastante dinero.

A: How does your husband feel?
B: He's not well.
A: What is his problem?
B: He suffers from earaches.
A: Why don't you consult a specialist?
B: Because we don't have enough money.

Grammar

PRESENT INDICATIVE OF THE IRREGULAR VERB *HACER*
(TO DO OR MAKE)

yo	**hago**	*I do, make*
él/ella	**hace**	*he/she does, makes*
Ud.	**hace**	*you do, make*
nosotros/nosotras	**hacemos**	*we do, make*
ellos/ellas	**hacen**	*they do, make*
Uds.	**hacen**	*you (pl.) do, make*

Grammar

IDIOMATIC EXPRESSION
WITH *HACER*

In Spanish we use an idiomatic expression with **hacer** to show that an action or a state of being has been going on in the past and continues in the present. It is equivalent to the English present perfect or the present perfect progressive tense. For this expression we use the verb **hace** plus *a specific time designation* plus **que** plus *another verb in the present tense.* For example:

Hace un año que estudio el español.   *I have been studying Spanish for a year.*

VOCABULARY

una hora   *an hour*

un cuarto de hora   *a quarter-hour*

una media hora   *a half-hour*

un día   *a day*

una semana   *a week*

un mes   *a month*

un año   *a year*

Oral practice

Answer the questions using the cues.

¿Cuánto tiempo hace que Ud. tiene dolor del oído?   *How long have you had an earache?*

Hace una hora que tengo dolor del oído.   *I have had an earache for an hour.*

1. ¿Cuánto tiempo hace que el paciente tiene dolor del oído?   • two hours
2. ¿Cuánto tiempo hace que la mujer tiene dolor del ojo?   • a half-hour
3. ¿Cuánto tiempo hace que la muchacha tiene dolor de la nariz?   • a day

4. ¿Cuánto tiempo hace que el joven tiene dolor de garganta?
5. ¿Cuánto tiempo hace que su padre tiene dolor de la boca?
6. ¿Cuánto tiempo hace que su mujer tiene dolor del cuello?
7. ¿Cuánto tiempo hace que su hijo tiene dolor de las encías?
8. ¿Cuánto tiempo hace que su abuelo tiene dolor de cabeza?
9. ¿Cuánto tiempo hace que su tío tiene dolor de la frente?
10. ¿Cuánto tiempo hace que su esposo tiene dolor de muelas?

- two days
- a week
- two weeks
- three weeks
- a month
- two months
- a year

Role playing

One student takes the role of the patient and reads the sentence aloud. Another student plays the doctor, who must find out how long the patient has been doing whatever it is. The patient then answers, giving a specific amount of time.

A: **Estudio el español.** — *I'm studying Spanish.*
B: **¿Cuánto tiempo hace que Ud. estudia el español?** — *How long have you been studying Spanish?*
A: **Hace dos semanas que estudio el español.** — *I have been studying Spanish for two weeks.*

1. Tomo la medicina.
2. Tengo dolor del estómago.
3. Siento dolor en la boca.
4. Vivo en esta calle.
5. Siento dolor en los ojos.
6. Tomo el jarabe.
7. Tengo dolor de cabeza.
8. Siento dolor en la frente.
9. Consulto con el especialista.
10. Tomo las píldoras.
11. Trabajo en la clínica.
12. Sufro de los nervios.
13. Estudio la medicina.
14. Preparo la receta.
15. Hago las camas.

OTHER IDIOMATIC EXPRESSIONS
USING *HACER*

Hacer, which normally means *to do* or *to make,* can be used in combination with a number of nouns to express actions normally expressed directly by verbs. For example, the verb **viajar** (*to travel*) can be replaced with **hacer un viaje** (*to make a trip*). In some cases, verbs other than *to do* or *to make* might be used in English (just as many people would say to *take* a trip).

hacer el análisis de la orina   *to do the urinalysis*
hacer un urinálisis   *to do a urinalysis*
hacer un análisis de la sangre   *to do a blood analysis*
hacer daño   *to do harm*
hacerse daño   *to harm oneself*
hacer los ejercicios   *to do exercises*
hacer el examen médico, el reconocimiento médico   *to perform an examination*

hacer gárgaras   *to gargle*
hacer la maleta   *to pack a suitcase*
hacer una pregunta   *to ask a question*
hacer un puño   *to make a fist*
hacer una radiografía   *to take an X-ray*
hacer el trabajo   *to work*
hacer una visita   *to make a visit*

Oral practice

Answer the questions with complete sentences.

1. ¿Hace el análisis de sangre el técnico?
2. ¿Hace el urinálisis el hombre?
3. ¿Hace el examen la doctora?
4. ¿Hace la maleta el paciente?
5. ¿Hace un puño el hombre?
6. ¿Hacen los ejercicios los muchachos?
7. ¿Hacen las preguntas los especialistas?
8. ¿Hace el trabajo la mujer?
9. ¿Hace el viaje el hombre?
10. ¿Hacen las radiografías los técnicos?

Conversations

A: ¿Cuánto tiempo tiene que quedarse mi padre en el hospital?
B: Una semana más o menos.
A: ¿Por qué?
B: Los técnicos tienen que hacer algunos análisis.
A: ¿Qué análisis tienen que hacer hoy?

B: Creo que hacen un análisis de la orina y otro de sangre.

A: How long does my father have to remain in the hospital?
B: A week more or less.
A: Why?
B: The technicians have to do some analyses.
A: What analyses do they have to do today?
B: I think that they are going to do an analysis of the urine and another of the blood.

A: ¿Cuánto tiempo hace que tiene la garganta irritada?
B: Hace dos días.
A: ¿Qué hace Ud. para el dolor?
B: Hago gárgaras con agua con sal.
A: ¿Alivia el dolor?
B: Sí, después de hacer las gárgaras, me siento mejor.

A: How long have you had a sore throat?
B: For two days.
A: What are you doing for the pain?
B: I gargle with salt water.
A: Does it relieve the pain?
B: Yes, after gargling I feel better.

A: ¿Cuánto tiempo hace que sufre de los nervios?

A: How long have you been suffering from nerves?

B: Hace un año.

B: For a year.

A: ¿Por qué está nerviosa?

A: Why are you nervous?

B: Porque tengo muchos problemas.

B: Because I have a lot of problems.

A: ¿Qué problemas tiene?

A: What problems do you have?

B: Mi esposo no tiene trabajo. No tenemos dinero y los niños siempre pasan hambre.

B: My husband is out of work. We don't have any money and the children are always hungry.

Grammar

PRESENT INDICATIVE OF THE IRREGULAR VERB *DECIR* (TO SAY OR TELL)

yo	**digo**	*I say, tell*
él/ella	**dice**	*he/she says, tells*
Ud.	**dice**	*you say, tell*
nosotros/nosotras	**decimos**	*we say, tell*
ellos/ellas	**dicen**	*they say, tell*
Uds.	**dicen**	*you* (pl.) *say, tell*

Oral practice

Answer the questions using the cues.

1. ¿Quién dice la verdad?
   - la enfermera • los médicos • el hombre • las muchachas • yo

2. ¿Quién dice que tiene prisa?
   - nosotras • los técnicos • la policía • el dependiente • el cajero

Answer the questions with complete sentences.

1. ¿Dice Ud. la verdad?
2. ¿Dice el paciente que tiene dolor?
3. ¿Dicen los especialistas que es un caso grave?
4. ¿Dice la enfermera que la paciente se siente mejor?
5. ¿Dice la doctora que Ud. necesita descansar?

Conversations

A: ¿Qué dice Ud.?

A: What are you saying?

B: Tienen que hospitalizar a mi marido.

B: They have to hospitalize my husband.

A: ¿Por qué?

A: Why?

B: Porque necesita una operación.

B: Because he needs an operation.

A: ¿Es grave su condición?

A: Is his condition serious?

B: El médico dice que no, pero yo estoy muy preocupada. Mi marido tiene miedo del hospital.

A: ¿Cómo se siente Ud. hoy?
B: No muy bien.
A: ¿Qué dice la doctora de su condición?

B: Dice que estoy muy débil. No como bastante y necesito tomar vitaminas. Lo que es más, estoy muy deprimida.

A: ¿Tiene apetito?
B: El problema es que no tengo apetito.

A: ¿Qué dice el médico de su condición?

B: Dice que estoy mejor.
A: ¿Qué dice su familia?
B: Mi familia está muy contenta.
A: ¿Se siente Ud. mejor?
B: Sí, pero todavía estoy un poco débil.

B: The doctor says it isn't but I'm very worried. My husband is afraid of the hospital.

A: How are you feeling today?
B: Not very well.
A: What does the doctor say about your condition?

B: She says that I'm very weak. I don't eat enough and I need to take vitamins. What is more, I'm very depressed.

A: Do you have an appetite?
B: The problem is that I don't have an appetite.

A: What does the doctor say about your condition?

B: The doctor says that I'm better.
A: What does your family say?
B: My family is very happy.
A: Do you feel better?
B: Yes, but I'm still a little weak.

Grammar

PRESENT INDICATIVE OF THE IRREGULAR VERB *SALIR* (TO LEAVE)

yo	**salgo**	*I leave*
él/ella	**sale**	*he/she leaves*
Ud.	**sale**	*you leave*
nosotros/nosotras	**salimos**	*we leave*
ellos/ellas	**salen**	*they leave*
Uds.	**salen**	*you (pl.) leave*

Oral practice

Answer the questions using the cues.

1. ¿Quién sale del hospital?
   • la pediatra • el enfermo • el joven • las mujeres • el técnico

2. ¿A qué hora sale Ud. de su casa?
   • 7:30 • 8:15 • 9:25 • 10:35 • midnight

Answer the questions with an original response.

1. ¿Quién sale del cuarto de la paciente?
2. ¿Cuándo salen Uds. del hospital?
3. ¿Con quién sale el joven?
4. ¿Sale Ud. temprano?
5. ¿Sale Ud. del hospital mañana?

Answer the questions using the cues.

1. ¿Cuándo sale su madre del hospital?   • today
2. ¿Cuándo sale el paciente del hospital?   • the day after tomorrow
3. ¿Cuándo sale su hijo del hospital?   • in a week
4. ¿Cuándo sale el enfermo del hospital?   • on Monday
5. ¿Cuándo salen los pacientes del hospital?   • at three in the afternoon
6. ¿Cuándo sale el enfermero del hospital?   • on Saturday
7. ¿Cuándo salen Uds. del hospital?   • at nine in the morning
8. ¿Cuándo sale la mujer del hospital?   • on Tuesday
9. ¿Cuándo sale su esposo del hospital?   • in two weeks
10. ¿Cuándo sale la muchacha del hospital?   • in a month

Conversations

A: ¿Cuándo sale Ud. del hospital?
B: Salgo mañana.
A: ¿A qué hora sale Ud.?
B: Salgo a las nueve de la mañana.
A: ¿Cómo se siente Ud.?
B: Me siento bien.

A: When are you leaving the hospital?
B: I'm leaving tomorrow.
A: At what time are you leaving?
B: I'm leaving at nine A.M.
A: How are you feeling?
B: I feel very well.

A: ¿Cuándo tiene Ud. que salir para el hospital?
B: Salgo en una hora.
A: ¿Qué hace Ud. ahora?
B: Hago la maleta.
A: ¿Necesita Ud. algo más?
B: Sí, necesito mi cepillo de dientes.

A: When do you have to leave for the hospital?
B: I leave in an hour.
A: What are you doing now?
B: I'm packing my suitcase.
A: Do you need anything else?
B: Yes, I need my toothbrush.

A: El médico dice que su padre no sale del hospital hoy.
B: ¿Por qué?
A: Porque no está bien.
B: ¿Qué hace el médico?
A: Tiene que hacer algunos análisis.
B: Entonces, ¿cuándo sale mi papá?
A: Quizás en dos semanas.

A: The doctor says that your father is not leaving the hospital today.
B: Why?
A: Because he is not well.
B: What is the doctor doing?
A: He has to do some analyses.
B: Well, then, when is my father leaving?
A: Perhaps in two weeks.

Grammar

PRESENT INDICATIVE OF THE IRREGULAR VERB *VENIR* (TO COME)

yo	**vengo**	*I come*
él/ella	**viene**	*he/she comes*
Ud.	**viene**	*you come*
nosotros/nosotras	**venimos**	*we come*
ellos/ellas	**vienen**	*they come*
Uds.	**vienen**	*you* (pl.) *come*

Oral practice

Answer the questions using the cues.

1. ¿Quién viene al hospital?
   - los médicos   • la enfermera   • mi padre   • la señora García   • yo

2. ¿Quién viene del hospital?
   - mi hija   • el hombre   • la doctora   • el señor Colón   • mis hermanos y yo

Answer the questions using the cues.

¿A qué hora viene el cura a la casa?   *When is the priest coming to the house?*
El cura viene a la casa a las tres de la   *The priest is coming to the house at three*
   tarde.   *P.M.*

1. ¿A qué hora viene Ud. al hospital?   • 4:30 P.M.
2. ¿A qué hora viene el médico al hospital?   • 7:00 A.M.
3. ¿A qué hora vienen Uds. al hospital?   • 10:30 A.M.
4. ¿A qué hora vienen sus hijos al hospital?   • 12:00 noon
5. ¿A qué hora viene su madre al hospital?   • 7:45 P.M.
6. ¿Cuándo viene la enfermera al hospital?   • 8:00 A.M.
7. ¿Cuándo vienen los médicos al hospital?   • 9:45 A.M.
8. ¿Cuándo viene la mujer al hospital?   • 3:25 P.M.
9. ¿Cuándo viene el enfermo al hospital?   • 2:00 P.M.
10. ¿Cuándo vienen sus abuelos al hospital?   • 11:00 A.M.

Conversations

A: ¿Con quién viene la doctora?
B: Viene con el especialista.
A: ¿Por qué?
B: Porque necesitan otra opinión.
A: ¿Por qué necesitan otra opinión?
B: Tienen que decidir si la operación es
   necesaria o no.

A: With whom is the doctor coming?
B: She's coming with the specialist.
A: Why?
B: Because they need another opinion.
A: Why do they need another opinion?
B: They have to decide whether the
   operation is necessary or not.

A: ¿A qué hora viene su marido al hospital?
B: Viene a las dos.
A: ¿Viene solo?
B: No, viene con mi hija mayor.

A: ¿Cuándo salen del hospital?
A: Salen a las tres de la tarde.

A: ¿Quién viene a visitar al paciente?
B: Vienen sus hijos y su nieto.
A: ¿Cuándo vienen?
B: Vienen a las dos de la tarde.
A: ¿Es su primera visita?
B: No, es su tercera visita en una semana.

A: At what time is your husband coming to the hospital?
B: He's coming at two.
A: Is he coming alone?
B: No, he's coming with my oldest daughter.

A: When are they leaving the hospital?
B: They are leaving at three P.M.

A: Who is coming to visit the patient?
B: His sons and grandson are coming.
A: When are they coming?
B: They're coming at two P.M.
A: Is it their first visit?
B: No, it is their third visit in a week.

Written practice

Translate the sentences into Spanish.

1. The patient is leaving the hospital tomorrow.
2. The technician is doing the analyses in the laboratory.
3. The patient in room thirty-two is very upset.
4. That man has a pain in his left ear.
5. Her children are coming to the hospital at eight.
6. How long have you had the pain?
7. What are you doing for your sore throat?
8. The doctor says that his condition isn't serious.
9. The nurses are coming now.
10. The therapist says that I must do the exercises.
11. My son has a pain in his right eye.
12. He has been studying English for a year.
13. We believe that he is telling the truth.
14. The specialist says that he needs an operation.
15. When are you leaving for the hospital?

Dialogue

VECINA: ¿Cómo está su abuelo?
NIETA: No se siente bien. Creo que tiene fiebre. El médico viene pronto.
MÉDICO: Buenos días, señora. ¿Dónde está su abuelo?
NIETA: Está en su cuarto, por aquí, doctor.
MÉDICO: Buenos días, señor. ¿Cómo se siente Ud. hoy?
ABUELO: Me siento muy mal. Tengo escalofríos.

MÉDICO: ¿Tiene Ud. dolor de cabeza?

ABUELO: Sí, tengo un dolor de cabeza muy fuerte.

MÉDICO: ¿Tiene Ud. dolor del estómago?

ABUELO: Sí, también tengo dolor del estómago.

MÉDICO: ¿Tiene Ud. diarrea o náuseas?

ABUELO: Tengo diarrea pero náuseas no.

MÉDICO: ¿Tiene Ud. dolor de la garganta?

ABUELO: Sí, tengo dolor de la garganta y además tengo mucha flema.

MÉDICO: ¿Cuánto tiempo hace que Ud. se siente así?

ABUELO: Hace dos días.

MÉDICO: Ud. tiene fiebre y la presión arterial está un poco alta. Tiene un virus con irritación en la garganta.

ABUELO: ¿Qué debo hacer, doctor?

MÉDICO: Receto un antibiótico que Ud. debe tomar cada seis horas. Debe tomar muchos líquidos y descansar mucho. Si se siente mejor en una semana, debe venir a mi consultorio. En todo caso, debe llamar por teléfono en un par de días.

ABUELO: ¿Es eso todo, doctor?

MÉDICO: Sí, Ud. es muy fuerte y su nieta está aquí para cuidar a Ud.

ABUELO: Muchas gracias, doctor.

MÉDICO: De nada, señor. Hasta pronto.

VOCABULARY

el vecino,-a neighbor
la fiebre fever
pronto soon
el cuarto room
por aquí through here, around here
los escalofríos chills
la diarrea diarrhea
las náuseas nausea
además besides, in addition
la flema phlegm
así so, this way, like this

la presión arterial blood pressure
alto,-a high
el virus virus
la irritación irritation
el antibiótico antibiotic
tomar to take
cada each, every
antes de before
el consultorio doctor's office
fuerte strong
cuidar to take care of

NEIGHBOR: How is your grandfather?

GRANDDAUGHTER: He's not feeling well. I think he has a fever. The doctor is coming soon.

DOCTOR: Good morning, ma'am. Where is your grandfather?

GRANDDAUGHTER: He's in his room, this way, doctor.

DOCTOR: Good morning, sir. How are you feeling?

GRANDFATHER: I feel very sick. I have chills.

DOCTOR: Do you have a headache?

GRANDFATHER: Yes, I have a very bad headache.

DOCTOR: Do you have a stomachache?

GRANDFATHER: Yes, I also have a stomachache.

DOCTOR:	Do you have diarrhea or nausea?
GRANDFATHER:	I have diarrhea but not nausea.
DOCTOR:	Do you have pain in your throat?
GRANDFATHER:	Yes, I have pain in my throat and I also have a lot of phlegm.
DOCTOR:	How long have you been feeling like this?
GRANDFATHER:	For two days.
DOCTOR:	You have a fever and your blood pressure is a little high. You have a virus and a sore throat.
GRANDFATHER:	What should I do, doctor?
DOCTOR:	I'm prescribing an antibiotic which you should take every six hours. You should drink a lot of fluids and get a lot of rest. If you feel better in a week, you should come to my office. In any case, you should call in a couple of days.
GRANDFATHER:	Is that all, doctor?
DOCTOR:	Yes, you are very strong and your granddaughter is here to take care of you.
GRANDFATHER:	Thank you very much, doctor.
DOCTOR:	You are welcome, sir. See you soon.

QUESTIONS ON DIALOGUE

1. ¿Dónde está el abuelo?
2. ¿Cómo se siente?
3. ¿Qué tiene?
4. ¿Qué otros síntomas tiene?
5. ¿Cuánto tiempo hace que se siente mal?
6. ¿Cuál es el diagnóstico del médico?
7. ¿Qué receta el médico?
8. ¿Qué debe hacer el abuelo?
9. ¿Qué debe hacer la nieta?
10. ¿Cuándo debe el abuelo llamar al médico?

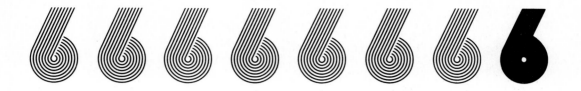

Vocabulary

THE TRUNK/EL TRONCO

la clavícula	*collar bone*	**el ombligo**	*navel*
el hombro	*shoulder*	**las caderas**	*hips*
la escápula	*shoulder blade*	**la pelvis**	*pelvis*
el omóplato	*shoulder blade*	**los órganos genitales**	*genitals*
los senos	*bosom*	**el pene**	*penis*
el pecho	*breast, chest*	**el miembro**	*penis*
el esternón	*breastbone*	**la vagina**	*vagina*
el tórax	*chest*	**el muslo**	*thigh*
el diafragma	*diaphragm*	**las entrepiernas**	*crotch*
las costillas	*ribs*	**la espalda**	*back*
la cintura	*waist*	**la columna vertebral**	*spinal column*
el abdomen	*abdomen*	**la nalga**	*buttocks*
el vientre	*abdomen*	**el ano**	*anus*
la barriga	*belly*	**el recto**	*rectum*

Oral practice

Answer the questions.

1. ¿Tiene Ud. dolor en el pecho?
2. ¿Tiene Ud. dolor en las costillas?
3. ¿Tiene Ud. dolor en el vientre?
4. ¿Tiene Ud. dolor de espalda?
5. ¿Tiene Ud. dolor de cintura?
6. ¿Tiene Ud. dolor en la vagina?
7. ¿Tiene Ud. dolor en el pene?
8. ¿Tiene Ud. dolor en la barriga?
9. ¿Tiene Ud. dolor en los senos?
10. ¿Tiene Ud. dolor en el muslo?

Answer the questions by following the model.

¿Cuánto tiempo hace que Ud. siente dolor en el pecho?	*How long have you felt pain in your chest?*
Hace un día que siento dolor en el pecho.	*I've felt pain in my chest for a day.*

1. ¿Cuánto tiempo hace que la paciente siente dolor en los senos?
2. ¿Cuánto tiempo hace que su madre siente dolor en las costillas?
3. ¿Cuánto tiempo hace que los pacientes sienten dolor en la barriga?
4. ¿Cuánto tiempo hace que su hijo siente dolor de espalda?
5. ¿Cuánto tiempo hace que la mujer siente dolor en la vagina?

Vocabulary

THE MONTHS OF THE YEAR/LOS MESES DEL AÑO

enero	*January*	**julio**	*July*
febrero	*February*	**agosto**	*August*
marzo	*March*	**septiembre**	*September*
abril	*April*	**octubre**	*October*
mayo	*May*	**noviembre**	*November*
junio	*June*	**diciembre**	*December*

Role playing

One student takes the role of the doctor and asks the student playing the patient where he/she is in pain. The patient responds mentioning a part of the trunk from the vocabulary list at the beginning of the unit. The doctor then asks how long the patient has been in pain. The patient responds giving a month of the year.

A: **¿Dónde tiene Ud. dolor?**	*Where are you in pain?*
B: **Tengo dolor del estómago (espalda, hombro, etc.).**	*I have a stomachache (backache, pain in my shoulder, etc.).*
A: **¿Desde cuándo tiene Ud. dolor del estómago (espalda, hombro, etc.)?**	*Since when have you had the stomachache (backache, pain in your shoulder, etc.)?*
B: **Desde enero (febrero, marzo, etc.).**	*Since January (February, March, etc.).*

Grammar

DIRECT OBJECT PRONOUNS

A direct object is a person or thing that receives the direct action of the verb. In the sentence *The student is buying the book,* the word *book* is the direct object of the sentence. The direct object pronouns replace direct object nouns: *The student is buying it.* Here is a list of the direct object pronouns:

	SINGULAR		PLURAL
me	*me*	**nos**	*us*
le	*you* (masc.), *him*		
lo	*you* (masc.), *him, it* (masc.)	**los**	*you* (masc.), *them* (masc.)
la	*you* (fem.), *her, it* (fem.)	**las**	*you* (fem.), *them* (fem.)

Direct object pronouns are placed before the conjugated verb. For example:

La joven bebe *el jugo*.	*The girl is drinking the juice.*
La joven *lo* bebe.	*The girl is drinking it.*
El niño lee *los libros*.	*The child is reading the books.*
El niño *los* lee.	*The child is reading them.*
La paciente toma *la medicina*.	*The patient is taking the medicine.*
La paciente *la* toma.	*The patient is taking it.*
El farmacéutico prepara *las recetas*.	*The pharmacist is preparing the prescriptions.*
El farmacéutico *las* prepara.	*The pharmacist is preparing them.*

Since the direct object pronouns in the third person singular and plural forms can have different meanings, the prepositional phrases **a él, a ella, a Ud., a ellos, a ellas,** and **a Uds.** may be used for clarity. They are usually placed directly after the verb.

La enfermera baña al paciente.	*The nurse is bathing the patient.*
La enfermera *lo* baña *a él*.	*The nurse is bathing him.*
La enfermera baña a los pacientes.	*The nurse is bathing the patients.*
La enfermera *los* baña *a ellos*.	*The nurse is bathing them.*

When direct object pronouns are used with an infinitive, they are attached to it. For example:

Debo tomar *la medicina*.	*I should take the medicine.*
Debo tomar*la*.	*I should take it.*

Oral practice

Replace the italicized direct object nouns with pronouns and make all other necessary changes.

La paciente toma *las píldoras*.	*The patient is taking the pills.*
La paciente *las* toma.	*The patient is taking them.*

1. Mi madre compra *los regalos*.
2. El médico analiza *el problema*.

3. Aceptamos *los cheques*.
4. Venden *la medicina*.
5. Recibimos *los paquetes*.
6. Necesito comprar *el jarabe*.
7. El farmacéutico prepara *las recetas*.
8. La doctora cura a *la paciente*.
9. La niña llama *al enfermero*.
10. Debo escribir *la carta*.
11. Tengo que visitar a *mi hijo*.
12. Comprendemos *la lección*.
13. Los técnicos hacen *los análisis*.
14. La mujer tiene que llenar *la receta*.
15. La paciente lee *la etiqueta*.

Grammar

INDIRECT OBJECT PRONOUNS

Indirect objects are persons or things that receive the action of the verb indirectly; that is, they answer the questions "to whom (what)?" or "for whom (what)?". Indirect object pronouns replace indirect object nouns. In the sentence *The student is buying the book for the teacher,* the word *teacher* is the indirect object of the sentence. The indirect object pronouns replace indirect object nouns: *The student is buying the book for her.* Here is a list of the indirect object pronouns:

SINGULAR

me *(to or for) me*
le *(to or for) him, her, it, you*

PLURAL

nos *(to or for) us*
les *(to or for) them, you* (pl.)

Indirect object pronouns are placed before the conjugated verb. For example:

Mi madre *me* compra la medicina. — *My mother buys me the medicine.*

El médico *nos* receta las píldoras. — *The doctor prescribes the pills for us.*

El farmacéutico *le* vende la medicina a él. — *The pharmacist sells him the medicine.*

Su padre *le* compra el jarabe para él. — *His father buys him the cough syrup.*

When there are two object pronouns involved, the indirect object pronoun precedes the direct object pronoun. For example:

Ella *me* receta la medicina. — *She is prescribing the medicine for me.*
Ella *me la* receta. — *She is prescribing it for me.*

Nuestra madre nos compra los regalos.	*Our mother is buying us the gifts.*
Ñuestra madre *nos los* compra.	*Our mother is buying them for us.*

Le and **les** must be replaced by **se** before **lo, la, los,** and **las.** For example:

La madre manda el paquete a él.	*The mother is sending the package to him.*
***La madre *se lo* manda a él.**	*The mother is sending it to him.*

Like the direct object pronouns, the indirect object pronouns are attached to the infinitive when they are used with it.

Mi madre tiene que comprarme la medicina.	*My mother has to buy me the medicine.*

When two object pronouns are attached to the infinitive, this form must be accentuated on the third syllable from the end. Thus:

La asistenta tiene que llevarme la comida.	*The aide has to bring me the food.*
La asistenta tiene que llevármela.	*The aide has to bring it to me.*

Oral practice

Replace the italicized direct and indirect object nouns with pronouns and make the necessary changes.

El técnico manda los resultados de los análisis al médico.	*The technician sends the results of the tests to the doctor.*
El técnico se los manda a él.	*The technician sends them to him.*

1. La madre compra *el regalo* para *su hijo.*
2. La mujer lleva *la comida* a *las pacientes.*
3. El muchacho manda *los paquetes* a *su abuelo.*
4. El farmacéutico vende *la medicina* al *cliente.*
5. El farmacéutico prepara *las recetas* para *los pacientes.*
6. La enfermera lleva *la medicina* al *paciente.*
7. La enfermera hace *la cama* para *el enfermo.*
8. Los técnicos hacen *los análisis* para *el médico.*
9. El hijo compra *las píldoras* para *su papá.*
10. Los técnicos llevan *los resultados* a *los especialistas.*

---

* In order to clarify to whom **se** refers, the prepositional phrase is added.

Grammar

PRESENT INDICATIVE OF THE REGULAR VERB *GUSTAR*
(TO PLEASE, TO BE PLEASING TO)

me gusta	*it pleases me*	**nos gusta**	*it pleases us*
le gusta	*it pleases him, her, you*	**les gusta**	*it pleases them, you* (pl.)

Gustar means literally *to please* or *to be pleasing to,* so it must always be accompanied by an indirect object pronoun. However, it is usually translated into English as *to like.* For example, **me gusta el libro** is literally *the book is pleasing to me,* but we would usually say *I like the book.*

The prepositional phrases **a mí, a él, a ella, a Ud., a nosotros, a ellas,** and **a Uds.** are used for emphasis or clarity. For example:

A él le gusta el libro.	*He likes the book.*
A ellas les gusta el libro.	*They* (fem.) *like the book.*
A Ud. le gusta el libro.	*You like the book.*
A mí me gustan los libros.	*I like the books.*

Oral practice

Change the sentences using the cues.

1. A mí me gusta el cuarto.
   - a ellos   • a Uds.   • a nosotros   • a ella

2. A él le gustan los regalos.
   - al paciente   • a las enfermeras   • a la mujer   • a mi padre

3. A mí me gusta trabajar.
   - al médico   • a los técnicos   • a la asistenta   • a mi hermano

Answer the questions in the affirmative and the negative by following the model.

¿Le gusta al paciente caminar?	*Does the patient like to walk?*
Sí, al paciente le gusta caminar.	*Yes, the patient likes to walk.*
No, al paciente no le gusta caminar.	*No, the patient doesn't like to walk.*

1. ¿Le gusta a Ud. el hospital?
2. ¿Le gusta a la paciente la comida?
3. ¿Le gustan a la muchacha los regalos?
4. ¿Les gusta a los médicos trabajar?
5. ¿Le gustan a la mujer las revistas?
6. ¿Le gusta al paciente el cuarto?
7. ¿Le gustan al hombre los periódicos?
8. ¿Les gusta a sus abuelos la casa?
9. ¿Le gusta al enfermo tomar la medicina?

10. ¿Les gusta a los pacientes hacer los ejercicios?
11. ¿Le gusta a su madre preparar la comida?
12. ¿Les gusta a Uds. estudiar el español?
13. ¿Le gustan al niño los libros?
14. ¿Les gusta a las enfermeras cuidar a los pacientes?
15. ¿Le gusta a Ud. la cerveza?

Conversations

A: Doctor, tengo tos con mucha flema.

A: Doctor, I have a cough with a lot of phlegm.

B: Tengo que examinarle a Ud.

B: I have to examine you.

A: ¿Es grave, doctor?

A: Is it serious, doctor?

B: Tengo que hacerle una radiografía.

B: I have to take an X-ray.

A: No me gustan las radiografías. Tengo miedo.

A: I don't like X-rays. I'm frightened.

B: No debe tener miedo. No es nada.

B: You shouldn't be frightened. It's nothing.

A: ¿Fuma Ud. mucho?

A: Do you smoke much?

B: Sí, dos paquetes al día.

B: Yes, two packs a day.

A: No debe fumar tanto.

A: You shouldn't smoke so much.

B: Pero me gusta fumar.

B: But I like to smoke.

A: Su salud es más importante.

A: Your health is more important.

B: Sí, doctor, comprendo.

B: Yes, doctor, I understand.

A: Ud. tiene que comer más vegetales, señora.

A: You must eat more vegetables, ma'am.

B: No me gustan los vegetales.

B: I don't like vegetables.

A: Pero tiene que comerlos, señora; son buenos para la salud. Debe tomar leche también.

A: But you must eat them, ma'am, they're good for your health. You should drink milk also.

B: No me gusta la leche tampoco.

B: I don't like milk either.

A: Ésta es comida del hospital y tiene que comerla. ¿Por qué no le gusta?

A: This is hospital food and you must eat it. Why don't you like it?

B: Porque tiene mal sabor.

B: Because it tastes bad.

Grammar

PRESENT INDICATIVE OF THE IRREGULAR VERB *QUERER*
(TO WANT, TO WISH, TO LOVE)

yo	**quiero**	*I want*
él/ella	**quiere**	*he/she wants*
Ud.	**quiere**	*you want*

nosotros/nosotras	**queremos**	*we want*
ellos/ellas	**quieren**	*they want*
Uds.	**quieren**	*you* (pl.) *want*

Oral practice

Answer the questions by following the model.

¿Quiere Ud. trabajar en el banco?	*Do you want to work in the bank?*
Sí, quiero trabajar en el banco.	*Yes, I want to work in the bank.*
¿Quieren Uds. trabajar en el banco?	*Do you want to work in the bank?*
Sí, queremos trabajar en el banco.	*Yes, we want to work in the bank.*

1. ¿Quiere Ud. entrar en la oficina?
2. ¿Quieren Uds. estudiar el español?
3. ¿Quiere Ud. hablar con la enfermera?
4. ¿Quieren Uds. enseñar la medicina?
5. ¿Quieren Uds. analizar el problema?
6. ¿Quiere Ud. aceptar el regalo?
7. ¿Quiere Ud. vender la medicina?
8. ¿Quieren Uds. vivir en la ciudad?
9. ¿Quiere Ud. escribir la carta?
10. ¿Quiere Ud. beber el jugo?

Change to the singular.

1. Los pacientes no quieren comer.
2. Los hombres no quieren tomar la medicina.
3. Mis hijos no quieren salir del hospital.
4. Los pacientes no quieren consultar con la doctora.
5. Las mujeres no quieren bañarse.
6. Las enfermeras no quieren trabajar en la clínica.
7. Los médicos no quieren estar en el cuarto.
8. Mis hermanos no quieren comprar las píldoras.
9. Los técnicos no quieren aprender el español.
10. Mis hijas no quieren acostarse a las diez.

Conversations

A: Señora, ¿por qué está Ud. tan triste?
B: Estoy sola, doctor.
A: ¿No tiene Ud. familia?
B: Mi marido no está en la ciudad y mi hija está sola en casa. No quiero estar en el hospital.
A: Pero Ud. está muy débil.

A: Why are you so sad, ma'am?
B: I'm all alone, doctor.
A: Don't you have any family?
B: My husband isn't in the city and my daughter is all alone at home. I don't want to be in the hospital.
A: But you are very weak.

B: No es verdad. Estoy bien, doctor. Quiero salir de aquí hoy.

A: ¿Es Ud. la recepcionista del Doctor Harris?
B: Sí, señora, soy su recepcionista.
A: Quiero fijar la fecha para mi próxima cita con el doctor.
B: Está bien. ¿Cómo se llama Ud.?
A: Me llamo Carmen Mendoza.
B: ¿Quiere Ud. regresar en dos semanas?

A: Sí, cómo no, señorita.

A: Quiero ver al médico.
B: ¿Por qué, señora?
A: No me siento bien.
B: Pero Ud. está mucho mejor, señora.
A: No lo creo, enfermera. No es cierto. Quiero hablar con el médico.
B: El médico no está aquí ahora.

B: It's not true. I'm fine, doctor. I want to leave here today.

A: Are you Doctor Harris' receptionist?
B: Yes, ma'am. I'm his receptionist.
A: I wish to set the date for my next appointment with the doctor.
B: Very well. What is your name?
A: My name is Carmen Mendoza.
B: Would you like to return in two weeks?

A: Yes, of course, miss.

A: I want to see the doctor.
B: Why, ma'am?
A: I don't feel well.
B: But you are much better, ma'am.
A: I don't believe it, nurse. That's not true. I want to speak with the doctor.
B: The doctor is not here now.

Grammar

PRESENT INDICATIVE OF THE IRREGULAR VERB *PREFERIR* (TO PREFER)

yo	**prefiero**	*I prefer*
él/ella	**prefiere**	*he/she prefers*
Ud.	**prefiere**	*you prefer*
nosotros/nosotras	**preferimos**	*we prefer*
ellos/ellas	**prefieren**	*they prefer*
Uds.	**prefieren**	*you* (pl.) *prefer*

Oral practice

Answer the questions with complete sentences.

1. ¿Prefiere Ud. consultar con otro especialista?
2. ¿Prefiere el paciente quedarse en el hospital?
3. ¿Prefiere su madre llamar a otro médico?
4. ¿Prefiere la mujer comer temprano o tarde?
5. ¿Prefiere el paciente descansar ahora o hacer los ejercicios?
6. ¿Prefieren sus padres hacer el viaje esta semana o la próxima semana?
7. ¿Prefiere Ud. venir sola o con su esposo?

8. ¿Prefieren las enfermeras trabajar en esta clínica o en otra?
9. ¿Prefieren Uds. quedarse aquí o regresar conmigo?
10. ¿Prefiere Ud. comer aquí o en la cafetería?

Answer the questions by following the model.

¿Prefiere Ud. este cuarto o ése?   *Do you prefer this room or that one?*
Prefiero ése.   *I prefer that one.*

1. ¿Prefiere Ud. este regalo o ése?
2. ¿Prefiere Ud. este libro o ése?
3. ¿Prefiere Ud. esta revista o ésa?
4. ¿Prefiere Ud. este periódico o ése?
5. ¿Prefiere Ud. esta casa o ésa?

Conversations

A: Enfermera, no quiero quedarme en este cuarto.
B: ¿Por qué, señor?
A: Porque prefiero un cuarto privado.
B: Lo siento, señor, pero todos los cuartos privados están ocupados.
A: Pues, si no hay remedio me quedo aquí.
B: Muy bien, señor.

A: Nurse, I don't want to stay in this room.
B: Why, sir?
A: Because I prefer a private room.
B: I'm sorry, sir, but all the private rooms are occupied.
A: Well, if nothing can be done, I'll stay here.
B: Very well, sir.

A: ¿Cómo está Ud. hoy?
B: No muy bien.
A: ¿Por qué?
B: Porque mi especialista dice que necesito una operación. Prefiero tener otra opinión.
A: ¿Por qué no consulta Ud. con mi especialista? Es muy bueno.
B: Prefiero esperar un rato.

A: How are you today?
B: Not very well.
A: Why?
B: Because my specialist says that I need an operation. I prefer to have another opinion.
A: Why don't you consult with my specialist. He's very good.
B: I prefer to wait a while.

Grammar

PRESENT INDICATIVE OF THE IRREGULAR VERB *IR* (TO GO)

yo	**voy**	*I am going*
él/ella	**va**	*he/she is going*
Ud.	**va**	*you are going*

nosotros/nosotras	**vamos**	*we are going*
ellos/ellas	**van**	*they are going*
Uds.	**van**	*you* (pl.) *are going*

The verb **ir** is followed by the preposition **a.** For example:

¿Va Ud. a la clínica hoy?	*Are you going to the clinic today?*
¿Van Uds. al hospital?	*Are you going to the hospital?*

The verb **ir** plus **a** plus an infinitive means *to be going to* in the sense of planning to do something in the future. For example:

¿Va Ud. a trabajar?	*Are you going to work?*
¿Va Ud. a examinarme?	*Are you going to examine me?*

Oral practice

Change to the plural.

Él va a aceptar la decisión del médico.	*He is going to accept the doctor's decision.*
Ellos van a aceptar las decisiones de los médicos.	*They are going to accept the doctors' decisions.*

1. Él va a comer en la cafetería.
2. La enfermera va a trabajar en la clínica.
3. La paciente va a tomar la píldora.
4. Voy a examinar los resultados.
5. Ella va a visitar a su amiga.
6. La paciente va a entrar en la consulta del médico.
7. Mi hermano va a salir del hospital hoy.
8. Voy a ir al laboratorio ahora.
9. El técnico va a hacer el análisis hoy.
10. La pediatra va a cuidar al niño.

Answer the questions with complete sentences.

1. ¿Con quién va Ud. a la clínica hoy?
2. ¿Va Ud. a trabajar mañana?
3. ¿A dónde va Ud. después de comer?
4. ¿Cuándo va Ud. a tomar la medicina?
5. ¿Cuándo va Ud. a salir del hospital?

Conversations

A: ¿Por qué no está contenta?
B: Tengo dolor. No tengo visitas. Todo va mal.

A: Why aren't you happy?
B: I'm in pain. I don't have any visitors. Everything is going wrong.

A: Le voy a hacer un reconocimiento médico.

A: I'm going to examine you.

B: ¿Qué me pasa, doctor?

B: What's happening to me, doctor?

A: La presión arterial está alta. No es nada grave pero Ud. tiene que quedarse en el hospital unos días más.

A: Your blood pressure is high. It's nothing serious but you have to stay in the hospital for a few more days.

B: Tengo que llamar a mi marido para decirle lo que pasa.

B: I have to call my husband to tell him what's going on.

A: Doctor, ¿qué me pasa? ¿Por qué no me dice nadie cuándo me van a operar?

A: What's happening to me, doctor? Why isn't anyone telling me when they're going to operate?

B: Tenemos que hacer más análisis. No es posible hacer un diagnóstico definitivo sin los resultados de los análisis.

B: We have to do more analyses. It's not possible to make a definitive diagnosis without the results of the analyses.

A: ¿Cuándo me van a hacer los análisis los técnicos?

A: When are the technicians going to take the analyses?

B: Se los van a hacer a Ud. mañana por la mañana.

B: They're going to take them tomorrow morning.

A: ¿Son análisis de sangre, doctor?

A: Are they blood tests, doctor?

B: Sí, señora. Ud. no debe preocuparse. Mientras tanto, tiene que descansar. La enfermera le va a dar una píldora para dormir.

B: Yes, ma'am. You shouldn't worry. In the meantime, you must rest. The nurse is going to give you a sleeping pill.

A: ¿A dónde va Ud. hoy?

A: Where are you going today?

B: Tengo una cita con el médico.

B: I have an appointment with the doctor.

A: ¿Por qué? ¿No se siente bien?

A: Why? Aren't you feeling well?

B: Hace unos días que no me siento bien.

B: I haven't felt well for a few days.

A: ¿A qué hora va a salir?

A: When are you going to leave?

B: Voy a salir a las dos porque la cita es a las tres.

B: I'm going to leave at two because the appointment is at three.

Grammar

PRESENT INDICATIVE OF THE IRREGULAR VERB *SEGUIR* (TO FOLLOW)

yo	**sigo**	*I follow*
él/ella	**sigue**	*he/she follows*
Ud.	**sigue**	*you follow*

nosotros/nosotras	**seguimos**	*we follow*
ellos/ellas	**siguen**	*they follow*
Uds.	**siguen**	*you* (pl.) *follow*

Oral practice

Change the sentences using the cues.

Sigo las instrucciones del médico.　　*I'm following the doctor's instructions.*
La paciente sigue las instrucciones　　*The patient is following the doctor's*
del médico.　　*instructions.*

1. Seguimos las instrucciones de la doctora.
   ● los pacientes　　● mi hermana　　● el paciente　　● yo

2. La mujer sigue a la enfermera.
   ● mi hijo　　● los hombres　　● la muchacha　　● las pacientes

3. Sigo al técnico al laboratorio.
   ● mi hija y yo　　● nosotros　　● el niño　　● las muchachas

Answer the questions using the cues.

¿Cuánto tiempo hace que Ud. sigue　　*How long have you been following a*
una dieta especial?　　*special diet?*
Hace tres meses que sigo una dieta　　*I have been following a special diet for*
especial.　　*three months.*

1. ¿Cuánto tiempo hace que la paciente sigue una dieta especial?　● two weeks
2. ¿Cuánto tiempo hace que el hombre sigue una dieta especial?　● a week
3. ¿Cuánto tiempo hace que la muchacha sigue una dieta especial?　● six weeks
4. ¿Cuánto tiempo hace que Uds. siguen una dieta especial?　● five days
5. ¿Cuánto tiempo hace que los pacientes siguen una dieta especial?　● one month

Conversations

A: Ud. tiene que seguir mis instrucciones, ¿comprende?

A: You must follow my instructions. Do you understand?

B: Sí, doctor, comprendo.

B: Yes, doctor, I understand.

A: Si no las sigue, Ud. no se va a curar.

A: If you don't follow them, you will not get well.

B: ¿Es grave mi condición?

B: Is my condition serious?

A: No, señor, Ud. puede salir del hospital esta semana.

A: No, sir, you can leave the hospital this week.

B: Muy bien, doctor. Muchas gracias por su ayuda.

B: Very well, doctor. Thank you very much for your help.

A: Mi hermana sigue una dieta estricta.
B: ¿Por qué?
A: Porque el médico dice que tiene sobrepeso.
B: ¡Pero a ella le gusta comer tanto!
A: Sí, es verdad. Pero si no sigue la dieta, se va a enfermar.

A: My sister is following a strict diet.
B: Why?
A: Because the doctor says that she's overweight.
B: But she likes to eat so much!
A: Yes, it's true. But if she doesn't follow the diet, she's going to get sick.

Written practice

Translate the sentences into Spanish.

1. I have had a pain in my chest for an hour.
2. She has been suffering from headaches since February.
3. The nurse (*masc.*) has to bathe the patient.
4. The specialist is going to examine the patient.
5. The doctor (*fem.*) is prescribing some pills for me.
6. The technician is going to take an X-ray of my chest.
7. I don't like to exercise.
8. He's afraid of the hospital.
9. The nurse wants to learn Spanish.
10. I wish to speak with the receptionist.
11. The patient (*masc.*) has to go to the clinic today.
12. He is in pain and he is very nervous.
13. They (*fem.*) have to take more tests.
14. My mother has to stay in the hospital for a week.
15. The doctor will make a diagnosis soon.

Translate the sentences into English.

1. Esa mujer tiene dolor en el seno derecho.
2. El médico le receta el antibiótico ahora.
3. ¿Por qué no le gusta hacer los ejercicios?
4. Doctor, no quiero tomar esta medicina porque tiene mal sabor.
5. Vamos a examinarle a Ud. ahora.
6. Ud. no sigue las instrucciones de la doctora.
7. Tengo dolor de espalda.
8. La enfermera va a hacerlo.
9. El farmacéutico no quiere vendérmelas.
10. El paciente en el cuarto 32 no quiere comer.
11. ¿Por qué no quiere Ud. seguir la dieta?
12. ¿Qué recomienda el médico?
13. Me duele mucho el hombro izquierdo, doctor.
14. Vamos a hacer el análisis ahora.
15. La señora prefiere ir a casa con su hijo.

Dialogue

DOCTORA: Buenos días, señora Martínez. ¿Cómo se siente Ud. hoy?

PACIENTE: No muy bien, doctora.

DOCTORA: ¿Qué tiene? ¿Por qué está tan nerviosa?

PACIENTE: Hace seis meses que tengo un chichón en el seno derecho. Es grande y muy duro pero no tengo dolor. ¿Puede ser un quiste o un tumor?

DOCTORA: Ud. tiene que calmarse. Vamos a ver lo que tiene. Voy a examinarle los senos.

PACIENTE: Me tiene muy preocupada, doctora. Si es maligno, no quiero una mastectomía.

DOCTORA: Sí, es cierto, puedo sentir algo en el seno. Puede ser un fibroma pero no puedo hacer ningún diagnóstico ahora. Necesitamos hacer una mamografía.

PACIENTE: ¿Qué es una mamografía?

DOCTORA: Es una radiografía de los senos.

PACIENTE: ¿Es necesario hacer la mamografía?

DOCTORA: Sí, y cuanto antes. Si es algo grave, es mejor descubrirlo pronto. De esta manera, podemos tratar de ayudarle.

VOCABULARY

un chichón *a lump*
duro,-a *hard*
un quiste *a cyst*
un tumor *a tumor*
maligno,-a *malign*
una mastectomía *a mastectomy*
cierto *true*

un fibroma *a fibroma*
una mamografía *mammography*
cuanto antes *as soon as possible*
mejor *better*
de esta manera *in this way*
tratar de *to try to*
ayudar *to help*

DOCTOR: Good morning, Mrs. Martínez. How are you feeling today?

PATIENT: Not very well, doctor.

DOCTOR: What's wrong? Why are you so nervous?

PATIENT: I have had a lump in my right breast for six months. It is big and very hard but it doesn't hurt. Could it be a cyst or a tumor?

DOCTOR: You must calm down. Let's see what you have. I am going to examine your breasts.

PATIENT: I am very worried about it, doctor. If it is malignant, I don't want a mastectomy.

DOCTOR: Yes, it is true, I can feel something in your breast. It could be a fibroma, but I can't make any diagnosis now. We need to do a mammography.

PATIENT: What is a mammography?

DOCTOR: It is an X-ray of the breasts.

PATIENT: Is it necessary to do the mammography?

DOCTOR: Yes, and as soon as possible. If it is something serious, it is better to discover it early. In this way we can try to help you.

QUESTIONS ON DIALOGUE

1. ¿Cuál es el problema de la señora Martínez?
2. ¿Cuánto tiempo hace que tiene el chichón en el seno derecho?
3. ¿Cómo es el chichón?
4. ¿Tiene dolor la señora?
5. ¿Qué le hace la doctora a la señora?
6. ¿Qué puede ser el chichón?
7. ¿Por qué no puede hacer un diagnóstico la doctora?
8. ¿Qué necesita hacer la doctora?
9. ¿Qué es una mamografía?
10. ¿Por qué es necesario hacer la mamografía cuanto antes?

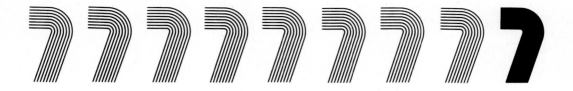

Vocabulary

THE UPPER EXTREMITIES/LAS EXTREMIDADES SUPERIORES

el brazo   *arm*
la axila   *armpit*
el codo   *elbow*
el antebrazo   *forearm*
la muñeca   *wrist*
la mano   *hand*
la palma de la mano   *palm*
el dorso de la mano   *back of the hand*

el dedo   *finger*
el (dedo) pulgar   *thumb*
el (dedo) índice   *index finger*
el (dedo) medio   *middle finger*
el (dedo) anular   *ring finger*
el (dedo) meñique   *little finger*
los nudillos   *knuckles*
las uñas   *fingernails*

Grammar

PRESENT INDICATIVE OF THE IRREGULAR VERB *DOLER* (TO HURT, TO ACHE)

me duele   *it hurts me*
le duele   *it hurts him/her/you*

nos duelen   *they hurt us*
les duelen   *they hurt them/you* (pl.)

me duele el brazo   *my arm hurts*
le duele el brazo   *his/her/your arm hurts*

nos duelen los brazos   *our arms hurt*
les duelen los brazos   *their/your arms hurt*

Because of the nature of its meaning, the verb **doler** is normally used only in the third person singular and plural, and in combination with indirect object pronouns. Notice that the subject of **doler** is that which hurts and the object is the person who feels the pain. The preposition **a** followed by the personal pronoun can be used for emphasis or clarity. For example, **A él le duele la mano.** (*His hand hurts.*)

Oral practice

Answer the questions first in the affirmative and then in the negative.

¿Le duele a Ud. el dedo?	*Does your finger hurt?*
Sí, me duele el dedo.	*Yes, my finger hurts.*
No, no me duele el dedo.	*No, my finger does not hurt.*

1. ¿Le duele a Ud. el brazo derecho?
2. ¿Le duele a Ud. el brazo izquierdo?
3. ¿Le duele a Ud. el codo derecho?
4. ¿Le duele a Ud. el codo izquierdo?
5. ¿Le duele a Ud. el antebrazo derecho?
6. ¿Le duele a Ud. el antebrazo izquierdo?
7. ¿Le duele a Ud. la mano derecha?
8. ¿Le duele a Ud. la mano izquierda?
9. ¿Le duele a Ud. la muñeca derecha?
10. ¿Le duele a Ud. la muñeca izquierda?
11. ¿Le duelen a Ud. los brazos?
12. ¿Le duelen a Ud. los codos?
13. ¿Le duelen a Ud. las muñecas?
14. ¿Le duelen a Ud. las manos?

VOCABULARY

agudo,-a	*sharp*	**quemante**	*burning*
constante	*constant*	**severo,-a**	*severe*
leve	*mild*	**sordo,-a**	*dull*
penetrante	*deep*		

Role playing

One student takes the role of the patient and reads the sentence aloud. Another student plays the doctor and asks how long the patient has been in pain. The patient answers specifying an amount of time. The doctor then asks what type of pain it is. The patient answers using one of the adjectives from the vocabulary list.

A: **Me duele el brazo derecho.**	*My right arm hurts.*
B: **¿Cuánto tiempo hace que le duele?**	*How long has it been hurting you?*
A: **Hace dos días.**	*For two days.*
B: **¿Qué clase de dolor es?**	*What type of pain is it?*
A: **Es un dolor constante.**	*It's a constant pain.*

1. Me duele el brazo izquierdo.
2. Me duele la mano derecha.
3. Me duelen los dedos.
4. Me duelen los nudillos.
5. Me duele el antebrazo derecho.

Vocabulary

THE LOWER EXTREMITIES/
LAS EXTREMIDADES INFERIORES

la pierna   *leg*   **el tobillo**   *ankle*
el muslo   *thigh*   **el pie**   *foot*
la rodilla   *knee*   **el talón**   *heel*
la rótula   *kneecap*   **la planta del pie**   *sole*
la pantorrilla   *calf*   **el empeine**   *instep*
la espinilla   *shin*   **los dedos de los pies**   *toes*

Oral practice

Change the sentences by following the model.

Tengo dolor en la pierna derecha.   *I have pain in my right leg.*
Me duele la pierna derecha.   *My right leg hurts.*

1. Tengo dolor en la rodilla izquierda.
2. Tengo dolor en la rótula derecha.
3. Tengo dolor en el tobillo derecho.
4. Tengo dolor en el talón izquierdo.
5. Tengo dolor en el empeine izquierdo.

Tengo dolor en las piernas.   *I have pain in my legs.*
Me duelen las piernas.   *My legs hurt.*

1. Tengo dolor en los muslos.
2. Tengo dolor en las rodillas.
3. Tengo dolor en los tobillos.
4. Tengo dolor en los talones.
5. Tengo dolor en los dedos de los pies.

Answer the questions using the cues.

¿Qué le van a operar a Ud.?   *What are they going to operate on?*
Me van a operar de la pierna   *They are going to operate on my left leg.*
 izquierda.

1. ¿Qué le van a operar al paciente?   • legs
2. ¿Qué le van a operar a su madre?   • right knee
3. ¿Qué le van a operar a su hermano?   • left kneecap
4. ¿Qué le van a operar a su padre?   • right foot
5. ¿Qué le van a operar a su esposo?   • toes

¿Qué le van a examinar a Ud.?
Me van a examinar los pies.

What are they going to examine?
They are going to examine my feet.

6. ¿Qué le van a examinar a su marido?
7. ¿Qué le van a examinar a su hermana?
8. ¿Qué le van a examinar a su mujer?
9. ¿Qué le van a examinar a su abuelo?
10. ¿Qué le van a examinar a su hija?

- legs
- left knee
- ankles
- heels
- calf

Conversations

A: ¿Tiene Ud. dolor?
B: Sí, me duele el brazo derecho.
A: ¿Es un dolor leve?
B: No, es un dolor agudo.
A: ¿Cuánto tiempo hace que le duele?
B: Hace tres días que me duele.
A: ¿Le duele otra parte?
B: Sí, me duele la muñeca derecha también.

A: Are you in pain?
B: Yes, my right arm hurts.
A: Is it a mild pain?
B: No, it's a sharp pain.
A: How long has it been hurting you?
B: It has been hurting me for three days.
A: Are you in pain anywhere else?
B: Yes, my right wrist hurts also.

A: ¿Qué le van a operar?
B: Me van a operar de la rodilla izquierda.

A: ¿Cuándo le van a operar?
B: Me van a operar el miércoles, el veinte de diciembre.
A: ¿Cuánto tiempo va a quedarse en el hospital?
B: Dos semanas.

A: What are they going to operate on?
B: They're going to operate on my left knee.

A: When are they going to operate?
B: They're going to operate on Wednesday, December 20th.
A: How long are you going to stay in the hospital?
B: Two weeks.

A: ¿Dónde tiene dolor?
B: Tengo dolor en la pierna derecha.
A: ¿Cuánto tiempo hace que le duele?
B: Hace una hora.
A: ¿Qué va a hacer para aliviar el dolor?

B: Voy a tomar un baño caliente.

A: Where does it hurt?
B: My right leg hurts.
A: How long has it been hurting you?
B: For an hour.
A: What are you going to do to relieve the pain?

B: I'm going to take a hot bath.

Grammar

PRESENT INDICATIVE OF THE IRREGULAR VERB *PODER* (TO BE ABLE, CAN)

yo	**puedo**	*I can*
él/ella	**puede**	*he/she can*
Ud.	**puede**	*you can*

nosotros/nosotras	**podemos**	*we can*
ellos/ellas	**pueden**	*they can*
Uds.	**pueden**	*you* (pl.) *can*

Like its English equivalent, this verb is always combined with an infinitive. For example:

Puedo hacer los ejercicios.	*I can do the exercises.*
Podemos salir ahora.	*We can leave now.*

Oral practice

Change the sentences using the cues.

1. Nosotros podemos comer ahora.
   • los pacientes   • su madre   • la muchacha   • su hijo

2. La paciente puede ir a la clínica hoy.
   • su abuelo   • nosotras   • Uds.   • el niño y yo

3. El muchacho puede hacer los ejercicios.
   • los pacientes   • el joven   • las mujeres   • yo

Answer the questions with complete sentences.

1. ¿Puede Ud. venir mañana?
2. ¿Puede el paciente caminar?
3. ¿Puede la enfermera bañarme ahora?
4. ¿Puede Ud. recetarme algo?
5. ¿Puede el técnico hacer los análisis?
6. ¿Puede el especialista hacer el diagnóstico?
7. ¿Pueden mis padres visitarme?
8. ¿Podemos salir del hospital ahora?
9. ¿Puede Ud. comprarme la medicina?
10. ¿Puede Ud. ayudarme?

Conversations

A: Doctor, ¿puede Ud. decirme cómo está mi padre? Mi marido y yo estamos muy preocupados. ¿Está muy enfermo?

B: No, señora, pero está muy débil y necesita un descanso. ¿Pueden Uds. cuidarle unas cuantas semanas?

A: No es posible, doctor.

B: ¿Por qué?

A: Mi marido y yo trabajamos de día. No hay nadie en casa todo el día. Mi padre no puede estar solo en casa.

A: Doctor, can you tell me how my father is? My husband and I are very worried. Is he very sick?

B: No, ma'am, but he is very weak and he needs a rest. Can you take care of him for a few weeks?

A: It's not possible, doctor.

B: Why?

A: My husband and I work during the day. There is no one at home all day. My father cannot be at home alone.

B: Pues, Uds. tienen que buscar a una enfermera especial. Ella puede quedarse en casa con su padre para velar su condición.

B: Well then, you need to look for a special nurse. She can stay at home with your father and watch over his condition.

A: ¿Puede Ud. salir del hospital hoy?
B: El médico dice que no.
A: ¿Por qué?
B: Dice que no estoy bien.
A: ¿Qué le va a hacer el médico para ayudarle?
B: Me va a recetar otro medicamento y los técnicos tienen que hacer más análisis.

A: Can you leave the hospital today?
B: The doctor says no.
A: Why?
B: He says that I'm not well.
A: What is the doctor going to do to help you?
B: He is going to prescribe another medication for me and the technicians are going to do more analyses.

Grammar

PRESENT INDICATIVE OF THE IRREGULAR VERB *VOLVER* (TO RETURN)

yo	**vuelvo**	*I return*
él/ella	**vuelve**	*he/she returns*
Ud.	**vuelve**	*you return*
nosotros/nosotras	**volvemos**	*we return*
ellos/ellas	**vuelven**	*they return*
Uds.	**vuelven**	*you* (pl.) *return*

Oral practice

Change the sentences using the cues.

1. Nosotros volvemos de la clínica.
   - las muchachas   - las enfermeras   - el médico   - la asistenta

2. Yo vuelvo a las tres de la tarde.
   - mis padres   - el especialista   - los cirujanos   - el hombre

3. Vuelvo con la enfermera.
   - los médicos   - la doctora   - el pediatra   - los padres

Answer the questions with complete sentences.

1. ¿A qué hora vuelve Ud. de la clínica?
2. ¿Cuándo vuelven sus padres de Puerto Rico?
3. ¿Vuelven Uds. con sus padres?
4. ¿Vuelve el técnico del laboratorio?
5. ¿Vuelven los médicos del cuarto del paciente?

Conversations

A: Mi marido vuelve hoy del hospital. Estoy muy nerviosa.
B: ¿Por qué?
A: Porque está muy enfermo.
B: ¿Por qué sale del hospital si no está bien?
A: Los médicos dicen que no pueden hacer nada por él. Es demasiado tarde.
B: ¿Qué tiene?
A: Tiene cáncer.

A: ¿A qué hora va a visitar a su marido?
B: A las dos.
A: ¿Qué le va a llevar?
B: Voy a llevarle la maleta porque mañana sale del hospital.

A: ¿Cuándo va a volver Ud. del hospital?
B: Vuelvo a las tres porque tengo que ir de compras.

A: My husband is returning from the hospital today. I'm very nervous.
B: Why?
A: Because he's very sick.
B: Why is he leaving the hospital if he's not well?
A: The doctors say that they can't do anything for him. It's too late.
B: What does he have?
A: He has cancer.

A: At what time are you going to visit your husband?
B: At two o'clock.
A: What are you going to bring him?
B: I'm going to bring him his suitcase because he's leaving the hospital tomorrow.

A: When are you going to return from the hospital?
B: I'll return at three because I have to go shopping.

Grammar

PRESENT INDICATIVE OF THE IRREGULAR VERB *MOVER* (TO MOVE)

yo	**muevo**	*I move*
él/ella	**mueve**	*he/she moves*
Ud.	**mueve**	*you move*
nosotros/nosotras	**movemos**	*we move*
ellos/ellas	**mueven**	*they move*
Uds.	**mueven**	*you* (pl.) *move*

Oral practice

Change the sentences using the cues.

1. Muevo los brazos.
   • el paciente   • su hija   • la joven   • nosotros

2. Muevo los dedos.
   • mi hijo   • la mujer   • los pacientes   • el niño

3. Muevo las piernas.
   - el anciano
   - los hombres
   - la paciente
   - nosotras

Answer the questions with complete sentences.

1. ¿Puede Ud. mover las piernas?
2. ¿Pueden Uds. mover los brazos?
3. ¿Puede el muchacho mover los pies?
4. ¿Puede su madre mover los dedos?
5. ¿Puede el paciente mover los dedos de los pies?

Conversations

A: No puedo mover las piernas. Tengo que usar una silla de ruedas.

A: I can't move my legs. I have to use a wheelchair.

B: ¿Qué dicen los médicos? ¿Va Ud. a quedarse paralizado?

B: What do the doctors say? Are you going to stay paralyzed?

A: Dicen que no pueden hacer nada.

A: They say that they can't do anything.

B: ¿No puede Ud. consultar con otros médicos?

B: Can't you consult with other doctors?

A: ¿Para qué? ¡Ellos van a decir lo mismo!

A: What for? They're going to say the same thing!

B: Ud. tiene que calmarse, señor. ¿Por qué dice estas cosas?

B: You must calm down, sir. Why do you say these things?

A: Porque no quiero vivir más. No puedo caminar.

A: Because I don't want to live anymore. I can't walk.

A: Señora, tiene que tratar de mover las piernas.

A: You must try to move your legs, ma'am.

B: Pero señor, no quiero moverlas.

B: But sir, I don't want to move them.

A: ¿Por qué?

A: Why?

B: ¡Porque me duelen tanto!

B: Because they hurt me so much!

A: Pero tiene que hacer los ejercicios, ¿comprende?

A: But you must do the exercises. Do you understand?

B: ¿Por qué?

B: Why?

A: Porque si no los hace, no se va a curar.

A: Because if you don't do them, you won't get better.

Grammar

PRESENT INDICATIVE OF THE IRREGULAR VERB *DORMIR* (TO SLEEP)

yo	**duermo**	*I sleep*
él/ella	**duerme**	*he/she sleeps*
Ud.	**duerme**	*you sleep*

nosotros/nosotras	**dormimos**	*we sleep*
ellos/ellas	**duermen**	*they sleep*
Uds.	**duermen**	*you* (pl.) *sleep*

Oral practice

Change the sentences using the cues.

1. El hombre duerme mucho.
   - yo   - nosotras   - la niña   - el joven

2. El médico duerme poco.
   - las enfermeras   - los técnicos   - el terapista   - la asistenta

3. El paciente duerme mal.
   - el enfermo   - la madre   - los pacientes   - mi abuela

Answer the questions with complete sentences.

1. ¿Duerme Ud. bien?
2. ¿Dónde duerme el hombre?
3. ¿Duermen Uds. mal?
4. ¿Duerme mucho el paciente?
5. ¿Duerme poco la enferma?

Conversations

A: Buenos días, señora. ¿Cómo está Ud. hoy?

B: Estoy muy preocupada.

A: ¿Por qué?

B: Es mi hijo. No duerme bien. Tiene pesadillas todas las noches.

A: ¿Tiene problemas en la escuela?

B: Sí, tiene miedo de los otros muchachos y muchachas. Tengo que consultar con el consejero de la escuela.

A: Good morning, ma'am. How are you today?

B: I'm very worried.

A: Why?

B: It's my son. He doesn't sleep well. He has nightmares every night.

A: Does he have problems at school?

B: Yes, he's afraid of the other boys and girls. I have to consult with the school counselor.

A: ¿Cuántas horas duerme Ud.?

B: Duermo seis horas.

A: Pero Ud. tiene que dormir por lo menos ocho horas.

B: No puedo dormir más de seis horas.

A: ¿Por qué?

B: Porque tengo dos empleos y no tengo el tiempo.

A: How many hours do you sleep?

B: I sleep six hours.

A: But you must sleep at least eight hours.

B: But I can only sleep six hours.

A: Why?

B: Because I have two jobs and I don't have the time.

Written practice

Translate the sentences into Spanish.

1. My arms and legs hurt me very much.
2. They are going to operate on my left knee tomorrow.
3. The orthopedist is going to operate on my arm.
4. How long do I have to stay in the hospital?
5. Can you prescribe something for the pain in my left arm?
6. Are you going to take more tests?
7. When are you and your husband leaving the hospital?
8. I can't move my legs.
9. He doesn't want to live any more because he can't walk.
10. The patient has to use a wheelchair.

Dialogue

PACIENTE: Señorita, estoy muy nerviosa.
ENFERMERA: ¿Por qué, señora?
PACIENTE: Porque mañana me van a operar de la rodilla derecha y creo que va a salir mal.
ENFERMERA: ¿Por qué dice Ud. eso, señora? Todo va bien.
PACIENTE: Creo que no voy a poder caminar más.
ENFERMERA: Eso no es cierto. Es una operación muy sencilla. No hay problema.
PACIENTE: Pero creo que voy a quedar coja. Mi hijo dice que esta operación puede tener complicaciones.
ENFERMERA: Cualquier operación puede tener complicaciones, señora. Pero Ud. necesita ésta.
PACIENTE: No quiero la operación. Quiero salir de aquí. Quiero ir a casa. ¿Puedo hablar con el médico?
ENFERMERA: Sí, por supuesto.
MÉDICO: ¿Qué pasa aquí? ¿Hay problema?
ENFERMERA: Esta señora tiene miedo de la operación.
MÉDICO: Tenemos que operarle, señora. Si no operamos, Ud. no va a poder caminar más. Además, es una operación muy fácil. ¿Por qué no se duerme ahora, señora?
PACIENTE: No puedo dormir.
MÉDICO: Ud. debe tomar una pastilla para dormir. Es inútil agitarse. ¿Está bien?
PACIENTE: Sí, doctor, muchas gracias.

VOCABULARY

salir mal *to turn out badly*   **pasar** *to happen, to occur*
caminar *to walk*   **fácil** *easy*
sencillo,-a *simple*   **además** *besides*

cojo,-a *lame, crippled*
la complicación *complication*
cualquier *any*
por supuesto *of course*

una pastilla para dormir *sleeping pill*
inútil *useless*
agitarse *to become upset*

PATIENT: Miss, I'm very nervous.

NURSE: Why, ma'am?

PATIENT: Because tomorrow they're going to operate on my right knee and I think it's going to turn out badly.

NURSE: Why do you say that, ma'am? Everything is going well.

PATIENT: I think I'm not going to be able to walk anymore.

NURSE: That's not true. It's a very simple operation. There's no problem.

PATIENT: But I think I'm going to be crippled. My son says that this operation can be complicated.

NURSE: Any operation can have complications, ma'am. But you need this one.

PATIENT: I don't want the operation. I want to leave here. I want to go home. Can I speak with the doctor?

NURSE: Yes, of course.

DOCTOR: What's going on here? Is there a problem?

NURSE: This lady is afraid of the operation.

DOCTOR: We must operate, ma'am. If we don't, you won't be able to walk anymore. Besides, it's a simple operation. Why don't you go to sleep now?

PATIENT: I can't sleep.

DOCTOR: You should take a sleeping pill. It's useless to become upset. All right?

PATIENT: Yes, doctor, thank you very much.

QUESTIONS ON DIALOGUE

1. ¿Por qué está nerviosa la señora?
2. ¿De qué parte del cuerpo le van a operar?
3. ¿Qué cree la señora?
4. ¿Qué dice su hijo?
5. ¿Qué quiere hacer la señora?
6. ¿Qué le dice la enfermera?
7. ¿Qué le dice el médico?
8. Por fin, ¿qué toma la señora?

QUESTIONS FOR DISCUSSION

1. Muchos pacientes tienen miedo de la cirujía. ¿En qué formas expresan este miedo?
2. ¿Cómo debemos tratar a una persona que tiene miedo de una operación? ¿Qué podemos decir a tal persona para calmarle?

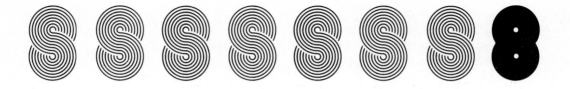

Vocabulary

THE ORGANS/LOS ÓRGANOS

el cerebro   brain
el oído   inner ear, hearing
las amígdalas   tonsils
los bronquios   bronchia
el corazón   heart
el pulmón   lung
el estómago   stomach
el intestino   intestine
el colon   colon
el riñón   kidney
el hígado   liver
el bazo   spleen
el esplín   spleen
el páncreas   pancreas

el útero   uterus
la matriz   uterus
el cuello uterino   cervix
la cerviz   cervix
el ovario   ovary
la vagina   vagina
los testículos   testicles
el pene   penis
el miembro   penis
el ano   anus
el recto   rectum
la vejiga   urinary bladder
la vesícula biliar   gallbladder

Oral practice

Answer these questions that a patient might ask.

PATIENT: **Doctor, ¿cuándo me van a sacar las amígdalas?**   *Doctor, when are you going to take out my tonsils?*

DOCTOR: **Le vamos a sacar las amígdalas mañana.**   *We are going to take out your tonsils tomorrow.*

1. Doctor, ¿cuándo me van a operar del cerebro?
2. Doctor, ¿tengo cáncer de la cerviz?
3. Doctor, ¿cuándo le van a operar a mi hijo?
4. Doctor, ¿qué puedo hacer para la infección del oído?
5. Doctor, ¿qué debo tomar para el dolor del estómago?

Cued situation

Pretend that you are a doctor interviewing patients in the following situations:

A. The patient has had an earache for three days.

1. Ask if it is a constant pain.
2. Tell him that you are going to examine his ears.
3. Tell him that he has to rest.
4. Tell him that he has to take some drops and some medicine that you are going to prescribe for him.
5. Ask him if he feels pain anywhere else.
6. Tell him that he must return in a week.

B. The patient has strong stomach pains.

1. Find out how long she has been in pain.
2. Ask her what she has been taking for the pain.
3. Ask her if she is constipated or if she generally suffers from constipation.
4. Ask her if she generally suffers from stomach pain.
5. Ask her if she eats well, has a good appetite.
6. Tell her that you need to take some tests.
7. Tell her that she must take the pills that you are going to prescribe.

Conversations

A: Le van a operar a mi hijo mañana.

A: They are going to operate on my son tomorrow.

B: ¿De qué le van a operar?
B: What are they going to operate on?

A: Le van a operar de las amígdalas.
A: They're going to operate on his tonsils.

B: ¿Quién le va a operar?
B: Who is going to operate?

A: Le va a operar el Doctor Menéndez, un cirujano muy bueno.
A: Doctor Menéndez, a very good surgeon, is going to operate.

A: ¿De qué le van a operar a Ud.?
A: What are they going to operate on?

B: Me van a operar del intestino.
B: They're going to operate on my intestine.

A: ¿Por qué?
A: Why?

B: Tengo una úlcera.
B: I have an ulcer.

A: ¿No puede Ud. tomar ningún medicamento?
A: Can't you take any medication?

B: No, porque la úlcera está muy grave.
B: No, because the ulcer is very bad.

A: ¿Tiene Ud. dificultad al respirar?
A: Do you have difficulty breathing?

B: De vez en cuando.
B: From time to time.

A: ¿Se cansa Ud. mucho?
A: Do you tire much?

B: Sí, me canso cuando estoy de pie por mucho tiempo.

A: ¿Fuma Ud.?

B: Sí, fumo dos paquetes al día.

A: Eso es malo. Ud. probablemente tiene fluido en los pulmones.

B: Yes, I get tired when I'm on my feet for a long time.

A: Do you smoke?

B: Yes, I smoke two packs a day.

A: That's bad. You probably have fluid in your lungs.

Grammar

PRESENT INDICATIVE OF THE IRREGULAR VERB *RECOMENDAR* (TO RECOMMEND)

yo	**recomiendo**	*I recommend*
él/ella	**recomienda**	*he/she recommends*
Ud.	**recomienda**	*you recommend*
nosotros/nosotras	**recomendamos**	*we recommend*
ellos/ellas	**recomiendan**	*they recommend*
Uds.	**recomiendan**	*you (pl.) recommend*

VOCABULARY

la cirugía   *surgery*
la clínica   *clinic*
el hospicio para ancianos   *nursing home*
el hospital   *hospital*

el medicamento   *medication*
el procedimiento   *procedure*
la terapia   *therapy*
el tratamiento   *treatment*

Oral practice

Change the sentences using the cues.

1. El especialista recomienda este procedimiento.
   • el médico   • el cirujano   • los especialistas   • la doctora

2. Recomendamos este hospicio para ancianos.
   • mi abuelo   • las enfermeras   • mis padres   • los médicos

3. Recomiendo esta clínica para los tratamientos.
   • nosotros   • el técnico   • los especialistas   • la pediatra

Answer the questions using the cues.

¿Qué recomienda el médico para la inflamación?

El médico recomienda esta medicina.

What does the doctor recommend for the inflammation?

The doctor recommends this medicine.

1. ¿Qué recomiendan los médicos para el dolor?   • these pills
2. ¿Qué recomienda el especialista para el dolor del oído?   • these drops

3. ¿Qué recomienda Ud. para mi padre?
4. ¿Qué recomiendan Uds. para este paciente?
5. ¿Qué recomienda la doctora para Ud.?

- these capsules
- these tablets
- these prescriptions

Conversations

A: Ud. tiene una infección de la garganta.
B: ¿Qué me recomienda, doctor?
A: Le recomiendo esta medicina que le voy a recetar.
B: ¿Es todo, doctor?
A: Además le recomiendo un descanso por un par de días.
B: Muy bien, doctor. Adiós.

A: You have a throat infection.
B: What do you recommend, doctor?
A: I'm recommending this medicine that I'm going to prescribe for you.
B: Is that all, doctor?
A: In addition, I recommend that you rest for a couple of days.
B: Very well, doctor. Goodbye.

A: ¿Qué recomienda el médico para su abuelo?
B: Recomienda un hospicio para ancianos.
A: ¿Por qué?
B: Porque mi abuelo ya no puede cuidarse.
A: ¿Por qué no puede vivir con Uds.? Pueden buscar a una enfermera especializada.
B: Es una buena idea. Tengo que hablar con mi esposo.

A: What does the doctor recommend for your grandfather?
B: He recommends a nursing home.

A: Why?
B: Because my grandfather can no longer take care of himself.
A: Why can't he live with you? You can look for a specialized nurse.

B: That's a good idea. I have to speak with my husband.

Grammar

PRESENT INDICATIVE OF THE IRREGULAR VERB *PENSAR* (TO THINK)

yo	**pienso**	*I think*
él/ella	**piensa**	*he/she thinks*
Ud.	**piensa**	*you think*
nosotros/nosotras	**pensamos**	*we think*
ellos/ellas	**piensan**	*they think*
Uds.	**piensan**	*you* (pl.) *think*

In addition to being used to describe the act of thinking, the verb **pensar** can be combined with other words to form other expressions. For example, when it is followed by the preposition **de** it means *to think about,* referring to opinion.

¿Qué piensa Ud. del hospital?   *What do you think about the hospital?*
Pienso que es un hospital bueno.   *I think that it's a good hospital.*

When **pensar** is followed by an infinitive it means *to intend to.*

> **Pensamos consultar con otro**
> **especialista.**
>
> *We intend to consult with another*
> *specialist.*

Oral practice

Change the sentences using the cues.

1. Pienso trabajar en esta clínica.
   - nosotros   • mi hermano   • las enfermeras   • el especialista

2. El enfermo piensa volver a casa.
   - los enfermos   • mi padre y yo   • la muchacha   • los jóvenes

3. Pensamos consultar con otro médico.
   - mi madre   • el paciente   • mis padres   • mi marido y yo

Answer the questions using the cues.

> **¿Qué piensa Ud. de las niñas?**   *What do you think of the girls?*
> **Pienso que las niñas son agradables.**   *I think that the girls are pleasant.*

1. ¿Qué piensa Ud. de las reglas del hospital?   • strict
2. ¿Qué piensa Ud. del técnico?   • competent
3. ¿Qué piensa el enfermero de los ejercicios?   • easy
4. ¿Qué piensan las enfermeras del médico?   • nice
5. ¿Qué piensan los padres del paciente del tratamiento?   • useless

Answer the questions with complete sentences.

1. ¿Piensan Uds. volver a casa pronto?
2. ¿Piensan Uds. hacer el viaje?
3. ¿Piensan Uds. ir a la farmacia para llenar las recetas?
4. ¿Piensan Uds. hacerme una visita pronto?
5. ¿Piensan Uds. operarme la pierna?

Conversations

A: ¿Qué piensa Ud. de la comida del hospital?

B: No me gusta.

A: ¿Por qué no le gusta?

B: Porque no se le echa sal.

A: Ud. tiene que seguir una dieta especial porque tiene la presión alta.

B: Sí, comprendo, pero pienso que es demasiado estricta esta dieta.

A: What do you think of the hospital food?

B: I don't like it.

A: Why don't you like it?

B: Because they don't put any salt in it.

A: You have to follow a special diet because you have high blood pressure.

B: Yes, I understand, but I think that this diet is too strict.

A:	Pensamos visitar a nuestro abuelo.	A:	We intend to visit our grandfather.
B:	¿Dónde está?	B:	Where is he?
A:	Está en un hospicio para ancianos.	A:	He's in a nursing home.
B:	¿Está lejos de aquí el hospicio?	B:	Is the nursing home far from here?
A:	No, está muy cerca.	A:	No, it's very near.
B:	¿Cuánto tiempo hace que está allí?	B:	How long has he been there?
A:	Hace dos años.	A:	For two years.

Grammar

THE PRESENT PROGRESSIVE TENSE

The present progressive tense is used to indicate that an action is in progress at the present moment. In Spanish it differs from the simple present in that it indicates that the action is taking place at the same time that is is being spoken about. The present progressive tense is formed by combining the present indicative of the verb **estar** and the present participle. In Spanish the present participle corresponds to the *-ing* form of the verb in English (*walking, talking,* etc.)

To form the present participle of an **-ar** verb, drop the final **-ar** and add **-ando** to the stem. To form the present participle of a regular **-er** verb, drop the final **-er** and add **-iendo** to the stem. To form the present participle of a regular **-ir** verb, drop the final **-ir** and add **-iendo** to the stem. For example:

tomar → **tomando**   *to take → taking*
comer → **comiendo**   *to eat → eating*
sufrir → **sufriendo**   *to suffer → suffering*

The following are examples of the present progressive tense:

Yo estoy hablando.	*I am speaking.*
Él/ella está hablando.	*He/she is speaking.*
Ud. está hablando.	*You are speaking.*
Nosotros/nosotras estamos hablando.	*We are speaking.*
Ellos/ellas están hablando.	*They are speaking.*
Uds. están hablando.	*You* (pl.) *are speaking.*

Oral practice

Change the sentences from the present to the present progressive tense by following the model.

Hablo español.	*I speak Spanish.*
Estoy hablando español.	*I am speaking Spanish.*

1. El técnico habla con la paciente.
2. El médico me llama.
3. El enfermo toma la medicina.

4. Tomamos el dinero.
5. Consulto con el especialista.
6. El médico analiza el problema.
7. El especialista cura a la mujer.
8. Ellos estudian el español.
9. Entramos en el cuarto del paciente.
10. El paciente dobla el brazo izquierdo.
11. Aprendemos a hablar español.
12. Bebemos el jugo.
13. El médico responde a la pregunta del paciente.
14. La mujer vende la ropa.
15. El niño corre por la casa.
16. Abrimos las ventanas.
17. La joven escribe las cartas.
18. El enfermo sufre mucho.
19. Su familia vive en la ciudad.
20. La enfermera abre las puertas.

Answer the questions with complete sentences.

1. ¿Quién está tomando la medicina?
2. ¿Quiénes están tomando las cápsulas?
3. ¿Quién está tomando las pastillas para dormir?
4. ¿Quiénes están tomando las píldoras?
5. ¿Quién está tomando las tabletas?

Answer the questions with complete sentences.

1. ¿Dónde está trabajando su marido?
2. ¿Dónde están viviendo sus abuelos?
3. ¿Con quién está consultando el paciente?
4. ¿Quién está hablando con el doctor García?
5. ¿Qué está bebiendo el paciente?

Grammar

IRREGULAR PRESENT PARTICIPLES

caer	*to fall*	**cayendo**	*falling*
creer	*to believe*	**creyendo**	*believing*
decir	*to say, to tell*	**diciendo**	*saying, telling*
dormir	*to sleep*	**durmiendo**	*sleeping*
leer	*to read*	**leyendo**	*reading*
morir	*to die*	**muriendo**	*dying*
seguir	*to follow*	**siguiendo**	*following*
sentir	*to feel*	**sintiendo**	*feeling*

Oral practice

Change the sentences from the present to the present progressive tense.

1. Decimos la verdad.
2. Los pacientes leen los periódicos.
3. El enfermo muere.
4. El paciente sigue las instrucciones del médico.
5. Dicen la verdad.
6. El niño duerme mal.
7. Sigo una dieta especial.
8. El farmacéutico lee la etiqueta.
9. Leemos las instrucciones de la doctora.
10. Las mujeres duermen.

Answer the questions with complete sentences.

1. ¿Está durmiendo la paciente?
2. ¿Quién está leyendo el periódico?
3. ¿Por qué están durmiendo sus hermanos?
4. ¿Quién está muriendo?
5. ¿Qué está diciendo el médico?

Written practice

Translate the sentences into Spanish.

1. What do you recommend for the pain?
2. He intends to work in this hospital.
3. He is taking the medicine now.
4. They are telling the truth.
5. He suffers from lung disease.
6. They are going to take out his tonsils tomorrow.
7. She has an ear infection.
8. The doctor is going to examine her ears.
9. The patient is dying.
10. He is following the doctor's instructions.

Dialogue

HIJO DEL PACIENTE: ¿Cuándo va el médico a examinar a mi padre?
RECEPCIONISTA: El médico está examinando a su padre ahora mismo.
HIJO DEL PACIENTE: ¿Cuándo va a terminar el examen?
RECEPCIONISTA: Debe terminarlo en unos momentos.
HIJO DEL PACIENTE: ¿Puedo hablar con el médico después?
RECEPCIONISTA: Sí, el médico va a hablar con Ud. después del examen.

más tarde

MÉDICO: Acabo de examinar a su padre.
HIJO DEL PACIENTE: ¿Dónde está?
MÉDICO: Está descansando en el consultorio. Quiero hacerle algunas preguntas a Ud.
HIJO DEL PACIENTE: Está bien, doctor.
MÉDICO: ¿Cuánto tiempo hace que su padre tiene estos síntomas?
HIJO DEL PACIENTE: Hace unos meses.
MÉDICO: ¿Está tomando algún medicamento?
HIJO DEL PACIENTE: No. No está tomando nada. ¿Qué tiene mi padre?
MÉDICO: Tiene diabetis.
HIJO DEL PACIENTE: ¿Es grave?
MÉDICO: Puede ser grave si su padre no sigue una dieta estricta.
HIJO DEL PACIENTE: Si es necesario, él va a seguir una dieta. ¿Hay algo más, doctor?
MÉDICO: Sí, le estoy recetando unas píldoras que él tiene que tomar según las instrucciones en la etiqueta.
HIJO DEL PACIENTE: Muchas gracias por todo, doctor.
MÉDICO: De nada, señor.

VOCABULARY

ahora mismo *right now*
después, después de *after, afterwards; after*
descansar *to rest*
seguir una dieta *to follow a diet*
las instrucciones *instructions*
la etiqueta *label*

PATIENT'S SON: When is the doctor going to examine my father?
RECEPTIONIST: The doctor is examining your father right now.
PATIENT'S SON: When is he going to finish the examination?
RECEPTIONIST: He should finish it in a few moments.
PATIENT'S SON: Can I speak with the doctor afterwards?
RECEPTIONIST: Yes, the doctor is going to speak with you after the examination.

later

DOCTOR: I have just examined your father.
PATIENT'S SON: Where is he?
DOCTOR: He's resting in the office. I want to ask you some questions.
PATIENT'S SON: Very well, doctor.
DOCTOR: How long has your father had these symptoms?
PATIENT'S SON: For a few months.
DOCTOR: Is he taking any medication?
PATIENT'S SON: No, he's not taking anything. What does my father have?
DOCTOR: He has diabetes.
PATIENT'S SON: Is it serious?
DOCTOR: It can be serious if he doesn't follow a strict diet.

PATIENT'S SON: If it's necessary, he is going to follow a diet. Is there anything else, doctor?

DOCTOR: Yes, I'm prescribing some pills that he has to take according to the instructions on the label.

PATIENT'S SON: Thank you for everything, doctor.

DOCTOR: You're welcome, sir.

QUESTIONS ON DIALOGUE

1. ¿Qué le pregunta el hijo del paciente a la recepcionista?
2. ¿Dónde está él médico?
3. Después del examen, ¿qué le pregunta el médico al hijo del paciente?
4. ¿Qué enfermedad tiene el paciente?
5. ¿Es grave su condición?
6. ¿Qué tiene que hacer el paciente para mejorarse?
7. ¿Qué le está recetando el médico para el paciente?

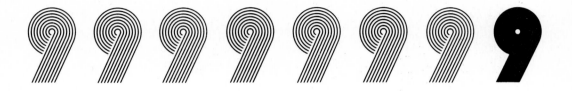

Grammar

PRESENT INDICATIVE OF THE IRREGULAR VERB *SABER* (TO KNOW, TO KNOW HOW)

yo	**sé**	*I know*
él/ella	**sabe**	*he/she knows*
Ud.	**sabe**	*you know*
nosotros/nosotras	**sabemos**	*we know*
ellos/ellas	**saben**	*they know*
Uds.	**saben**	*you (pl.) know*

The verb **saber** means *to know* in the sense of a knowledge of something factual, as in:

La recepcionista sabe donde está el médico.　　*The receptionist knows where the doctor is.*

This verb means *to know how to* when it is followed by an infinitive, as in:

Sabemos hablar español.　　*We know how to speak Spanish.*

Oral practice

Change the sentences using the cues.

1. Sabe hacer los ejercicios.
   - los pacientes　　● la muchacha　　● mi hijo　　● nosotras

2. Sé hablar español.
   - la enfermera　　● los médicos　　● el técnico　　● ella y yo

3. Sabemos hacer los análisis.
   - el técnico　　● la doctora　　● mi hermano　　● Uds.

Change the sentences to the singular following the model.

Los vecinos saben que el hombre maltrata a su hijo.	*The neighbors know that the man abuses his son.*
El vecino sabe que el hombre maltrata a su hijo.	*The neighbor knows that the man abuses his son.*

1. Los médicos saben que la joven se muere.
2. Sabemos que su padre está enfermo.
3. Los maestros saben que el niño está muy nervioso.
4. Los pacientes saben que la doctora viene pronto.
5. Las enfermeras saben que él tiene que tomar la medicina a las tres.

Answer the questions with complete sentences.

1. ¿Sabe su madre cuándo viene el especialista?
2. ¿Sabe Ud. dónde está la terapista?
3. ¿Sabe la psicóloga por qué está tan nerviosa la paciente?
4. ¿Saben Uds. dónde vive el hombre?
5. ¿Sabe la recepcionista dónde están los médicos?

Conversations

A: ¿Cuál es el problema?

B: El paciente en este cuarto no quiere comer. No sé qué hacer. ¡Está tan débil!

A: ¡Qué lástima! ¿Por qué no quiere comer?

B: Dice que está deprimido.

A: ¿Tiene visitas?

B: Creo que no tiene familia aquí. Vive solo.

A: Enfermera, ¿sabe Ud. dónde está el médico?

B: ¿Cuál es su problema, señor?

A: Quiero saber cuándo me van a operar.

B: El médico no está en el hospital ahora. Ud. tiene que esperar un rato.

A: ¿Sabe Ud. cuándo viene al hospital?

B: Viene pronto, señor. No se preocupe tanto.

A: What is the problem?

B: The patient in this room doesn't want to eat. I don't know what to do. He's so weak!

A: What a shame! Why doesn't he want to eat?

B: He says he's depressed.

A: Does he have any visitors?

B: I don't think that he has any family here. He lives alone.

A: Nurse, do you know where the doctor is?

B: What is the problem, sir?

A: I want to know when they're going to operate on me.

B: The doctor is not in the hospital now. You must wait a while.

A: Do you know when he's coming to the hospital?

B: He's coming soon, sir. Don't worry so much.

Grammar

PRESENT INDICATIVE OF THE IRREGULAR VERB *CONOCER* (TO KNOW, TO BE ACQUAINTED WITH, TO BE FAMILIAR WITH)

yo	**conozco**	*I know*
él/ella	**conoce**	*he/she knows*
Ud.	**conoce**	*you know*
nosotros/nosotras	**conocemos**	*we know*
ellos/ellas	**conocen**	*they know*
Uds.	**conocen**	*you* (pl.) *know*

Conocer is another verb that means *to know,* but it usually refers to people and is used to mean *to be acquainted with.* For example:

¿Conoce Ud. a mi padre?	*Do you know my father?*
Sí, conozco a su padre.	*Yes, I know your father.*

This verb also means *to know* in the sense of *to be familiar with,* as in:

¿Conoce Ud. el caso?	*Are you familiar with the case?*
Sí, conozco el caso.	*Yes, I'm familiar with the case.*

Oral practice

Change the sentences using the cues.

1. Conozco a su padre.
   - el médico • mi esposo y yo • la enfermera • los médicos

2. Ella conoce al técnico.
   - las especialistas • nosotros • mi abuelo • yo

3. Conocemos a la doctora.
   - mi madre • los hombres • mi hermana y yo • la muchacha

Answer the questions with complete sentences.

1. ¿Conoce Ud. al cirujano?
2. ¿Conocen Uds. al técnico?
3. ¿Conoce la paciente a este especialista?
4. ¿Conocen sus padres a este médico?
5. ¿Conoce la mujer a esta ginecóloga?

Conversations

A: ¿Conoce Ud. el caso?
B: Sí, conozco el caso. Se trata de un anciano que no quiere ingresar en un hospicio para ancianos.

A: Are you familiar with the case?
B: Yes, I'm familiar with the case. It has to do with an old man who doesn't want to enter a nursing home.

A: ¿Por qué?

B: Porque quiere seguir viviendo solo.

A: ¿Pero si ya no puede cuidarse a sí mismo?

B: No le importa. Dice que no quiere vivir en un hospicio porque para él, es una cárcel.

A: No conozco a nadie aquí. Me siento tan solo.

B: ¿Por qué no habla con los otros pacientes?

A: Porque son muy antipáticos.

B: ¿Por qué dice Ud. eso?

A: Es verdad. Hasta las enfermeras son desagradables.

B: Ud. está diciendo esto porque no se siente bien. ¿Por qué no trata de descansar un rato?

A: Why?

B: Because he wants to continue living alone.

A: But if he can't take care of himself anymore?

B: It doesn't matter to him. He says that he doesn't want to live in a nursing home because he considers it to be a prison.

A: I don't know anyone here. I feel so alone.

B: Why don't you speak with the other patients?

A: Because they're very unfriendly.

B: Why do you say that?

A: It's true. Even the nurses are unpleasant.

B: You're saying this because you don't feel well. Why don't you try to rest for a while?

Grammar

THE PAST PARTICIPLE AND THE PRESENT PERFECT TENSE

The present perfect tense is a compound past tense that is used to indicate an action or event that has taken place in the recent past. In Spanish the present perfect tense is formed by using the present indicative of the irregular verb **haber** (auxiliary verb meaning *to have*) and the past participle. In English the past participle usually ends in -ed or -en (*taken, eaten, suffered*). To form the past participle in Spanish of a regular **-ar** verb, drop the final **-ar** and add **-ado** to the stem. To form the past participle of a regular **-er** verb, drop the final **-er** and add **-ido** to the stem. To form the past participle of a regular **-ir** verb, drop the final **-ir** and add **-ido** to the stem. For example:

> **tomar** → **tomado**   *to take* → *taken*
> **comer** → **comido**   *to eat* → *eaten*
> **sufrir** → **sufrido**   *to suffer* → *suffered*

Here is the present perfect tense of the regular verb **hablar**:

Yo he hablado.	*I have spoken.*
Él/ella ha hablado.	*He/she has spoken.*
Uds. han hablado.	*You have spoken.*
Nosotros/nosotras hemos hablado.	*We have spoken.*
Ellos/ellas han hablado.	*They have spoken.*
Uds. han hablado.	*You* (pl.) *have spoken.*

Oral practice

Answer the questions by following the model.

¿Ha hablado Ud. con el médico?   *Have you spoken with the doctor?*
Sí, he hablado con el médico.   *Yes, I've spoken with the doctor.*

1. ¿Ha llamado Ud. al médico?
2. ¿Ha tomado Ud. las cápsulas?
3. ¿Ha consultado Ud. con el cirujano?
4. ¿Han aprendido Uds. el español?
5. ¿Han bebido Uds. el líquido?
6. ¿Han respondido Uds. a las preguntas de la recepcionista?
7. ¿Ha comido él?
8. ¿Han vivido ellas en Puerto Rico?
9. ¿Han sufrido ellos?
10. ¿Ha decidido ella ir al hospital?

Answer the questions with complete sentences.

1. ¿Ha tratado el médico de explicar la situación a la mujer?
2. ¿Han tenido Uds. problemas con sus padres?
3. ¿Ha sentido el paciente dolor en el abdomen?
4. ¿Han analizado el problema los médicos?
5. ¿Ha tomado Ud. las píldoras?

VOCABULARY

la náusea   *nausea*
los escalofríos   *chills*
tener eructos   *belching*
tener vómitos de sangre   *to vomit blood*
el gastritis   *gastritis*

la diarrea   *diarrhea*
los hemorroides sangrantes   *bleeding hemorrhoids*
las almorranas   *piles, hemmorrhoids*
el estreñimiento   *constipation*

Oral practice

Change the sentences from the present to the present perfect tense following the model.

Tengo problemas con los ojos.   *I have problems with my eyes.*
He tenido problemas con los ojos.   *I have had problems with my eyes.*

1. Tengo problemas con el oído.
2. El paciente tiene problemas con los dientes.
3. La mujer tiene problemas con la nariz.
4. Tengo problemas con las fosas nasales.
5. La muchacha tiene problemas con la garganta.

Vocabulary

COMMON SICKNESSES AND AILMENTS/ENFERMEDADES Y DOLENCIAS COMUNES

el dolor de cabeza *headache*
la jaqueca *headache*
la migraña *migraine*
las convulsiones *convulsions*
tener mareo *to be dizzy*
la calentura *fever*
la fiebre *fever*
las cataratas *cataracts*
el glaucoma *glaucoma*
el dolor del oído *earache*
la sinusitis *sinusitis*
la flema *phlegm*
tener catarro *to have a cold*

tener un resfriado *to have a cold*
estar constipado,-a *to have congestion*
resfriarse *to catch (to get) a cold*
la garganta irritada *sore throat*
la ronquera *hoarseness*
la laringitis *laryngitis*
la bronquitis *bronchitis*
la pulmonía *pneumonia*
la tuberculosis *tuberculosis*
las palpitaciones *palpitations*
el ataque de vértigo *dizziness*
la indigestión *indigestion*

Oral practice

Tengo hinchazón en el cuello. *I have a swelling in my neck.*
He tenido hinchazón en el cuello. *I have had a swelling in my neck.*

1. Tenemos hinchazón en las piernas.
2. La paciente tiene hinchazón en los pies.
3. Mi madre tiene hinchazón en los tobillos.
4. Los hombres tienen hinchazón en los brazos.
5. El niño tiene hinchazón en el ojo.

Sufro de jaqueca. *I suffer from headaches.*
He sufrido de jaqueca. *I have suffered from headaches.*

1. Sufrimos de cataratas.
2. El hombre sufre de glaucoma.
3. Mi tío sufre de inflamación del ojo.
4. Ellos sufren de dolores del oído.
5. El joven sufre de sinusitis.

Answer the questions in the present perfect tense.

1. ¿Ha tenido Ud. fiebre?
2. ¿Ha tenido Ud. convulsiones?
3. ¿Ha tenido Ud. mareo?
4. ¿Ha tenido Ud. náusea?
5. ¿Ha tenido Ud. escalofríos?

Change the sentences from the present perfect to the present tense.

1. He tenido los ojos inflamados.
2. Hemos tenido flema.
3. La enfermera ha tenido la garganta irritada.
4. El hombre ha tenido ronquera.

5. Mi marido ha tenido bronquitis.
6. Mi hermana ha tenido laringitis.
7. Las mujeres han tenido pulmonía.
8. Mi hermano y yo hemos tenido resfriados frecuentes.
9. Mi abuelo ha tenido tuberculosis.
10. Mi mujer ha tenido sinusitis.

Answer the questions in the present perfect tense.

1. ¿Tiene Ud. problemas con la respiración?
2. ¿Tiene Ud. dolor en la región del corazón?
3. ¿Tiene Ud. palpitaciones del corazón?
4. ¿Tiene Ud. ataques de vértigo?
5. ¿Tiene Ud. indigestión?
6. ¿Tiene Ud. dolor en el abdomen?
7. ¿Tiene Ud. eructos?
8. ¿Tiene Ud. vómitos de sangre?
9. ¿Tiene Ud. gastritis?
10. ¿Tiene Ud. diarrea?
11. ¿Tiene Ud. hemorroides sangrantes?
12. ¿Tiene Ud. almorranas?
13. ¿Tiene Ud. problemas con el páncreas?
14. ¿Tiene Ud. problemas con el hígado?
15. ¿Tiene Ud. problemas con la vesícula biliar?

Conversations

A: ¿Ha tenido Ud. problemas con el oído?
B: Ahora no, pero de niño sí.
A: ¿Ha sufrido de problemas con los ojos?
B: No, doctor, tengo muy buena vista.
A: ¿Ha tenido amigdalitis?
B: Sí, me han sacado las amígdalas.

A: Have you had problems with your hearing?
B: Not now, but as a child yes.
A: Have you suffered from problems with your eyes?
B: No, doctor, my vision is very good.
A: Have you had tonsilitis?
B: Yes, I have had my tonsils taken out.

A: ¿Ha sufrido de paperas de niño?
B: No, nunca he sufrido de paperas.
A: ¿Ha sufrido de sarampión?
B: Sí, he tenido sarampión.
A: ¿Ha sufrido de las viruelas locas?
B: No, no he sufrido de las viruelas locas.

A: Did you have the mumps as a child?
B: No, I've never had the mumps.
A: Have you had measles?
B: Yes, I've had measles.
A: Have you had chicken pox?
B: No, I haven't had chicken pox.

Grammar

IRREGULAR PAST PARTICIPLES

abrir	*to open*	**abierto**	*opened*
cubrir	*to cover*	**cubierto**	*covered*
decir	*to say, tell*	**dicho**	*said, told*
escribir	*to write*	**escrito**	*written*
hacer	*to do, make*	**hecho**	*done, made*
morir	*to die*	**muerto**	*died*
poner	*to put, place*	**puesto**	*put, placed*
ver	*to see*	**visto**	*seen*
volver	*to return*	**vuelto**	*returned*

Answer the questions with complete sentences.

1. ¿Han abierto Uds. las ventanas?
2. ¿Ha dicho Ud. la verdad?
3. ¿Ha escrito el médico la receta?
4. ¿Han hecho los pacientes los ejercicios?
5. ¿Ha muerto la mujer?

Change the sentences from the present to the present perfect tense.

1. Las enfermeras no dicen nada.
2. La doctora escribe la receta.
3. El paciente abre la puerta.
4. El médico examina a la mujer.
5. La paciente toma la medicina.
6. El especialista entra en el cuarto del paciente.
7. El técnico va a la cafetería.
8. El enfermero baña al paciente.
9. El cura viene pronto.
10. La señora me hace una visita.

Grammar

PRESENT INDICATIVE OF THE IRREGULAR VERB *PADECER* (TO SUFFER, TO BE AFFLICTED)

yo	**padezco**	*I suffer*
él/ella	**padece**	*he/she suffers*
Ud.	**padece**	*you suffer*
nosotros/nosotras	**padecemos**	*we suffer*
ellos/ellas	**padecen**	*they suffer*
Uds.	**padecen**	*you* (pl.) *suffer*

Padecer followed by the preposition **de** means *to suffer from.* For example:

La niña padece de corea.   *The child suffers from chorea.*

Vocabulary

CONTAGIOUS DISEASES/LAS ENFERMEDADES CONTAGIOSAS

la corea *chorea*	**la poliomielitis** *polio, poliomyelitis*
la difteria *diphtheria*	**la rubéola** *rubella, German measles*
la disentería *dysentery*	**el sarampión** *measles*
la escarlatina *scarlet fever*	**el tétano** *tetanus*
la fiebre amarilla *yellow fever*	**la tos ferina** *whooping cough*
la hepatitis *hepatitis*	**la tuberculosis** *tuberculosis*
la malaria *malaria*	**la tifoidea** *typhoid*
el paludismo *malaria*	**la viruela** *smallpox*
la meningitis *meningitis*	**las viruelas locas** *chicken pox*
las paperas *mumps*	

Oral practice

Change the sentences using the cues.

1. La mujer padece de hepatitis.
   - yo   • mi hermano   • mi tía   • nosotros

2. Mis hijos padecen de paperas.
   - mi sobrino   • mi hija   • la niña   • los niños

3. Los pacientes padecen de difteria.
   - el hombre   • yo   • las mujeres   • mi marido

Answer the questions with complete sentences.

1. ¿Ha padecido Ud. de corea?
2. ¿Ha padecido algún miembro de su familia de hepatitis?
3. ¿Ha padecido su hijo de escarlatina?
4. ¿Han padecido Uds. de malaria?
5. ¿Ha padecido el joven de disentería?

Written practice

Translate the sentences into Spanish.

1. They are going to remove her tonsils the day after tomorrow.
2. He often suffers from stomach pain.
3. He has taken the pills prescribed by the specialist.
4. She has spoken with the surgeon.

5. The patient has suffered a lot.
6. I have had problems with my eyes.
7. The patient has dysentery.
8. We need another opinion.
9. My son has already had the mumps.
10. He has never had the measles.

Translate the sentences into English.

1. El técnico ha hecho los análisis.
2. El paciente ha padecido de corea.
3. La doctora ha escrito la receta.
4. No hemos consultado con otros cirujanos.
5. Mi hijo padece de los riñones.
6. La enfermera ha abierto las ventanas.
7. Mi hijo padece de rubéola.
8. Su abuelo ha padecido de un ataque al corazón.
9. El paciente ha tomado la medicina.
10. No, nunca he padecido de la fiebre amarilla.

Reading

La enfermera entra en el cuarto del paciente para saber si se siente mejor. El paciente ha tenido una operación. Le han sacado cálculos de los riñones. La operación ha salido muy bien y el paciente se siente bien. De todas maneras, la enfermera le toma la temperatura y la presión arterial y le registra el pulso. Todo está normal. El paciente está mucho mejor.

Luego entra el especialista en el cuarto del paciente. Consulta el caso con la enfermera. Deciden que el paciente puede salir del hospital dentro de una semana.

VOCABULARY

el cuarto	*room*	**de todas maneras**	*in any case*
mejor	*better*	**la presión arterial**	*blood pressure*
sacar	*to remove, to take out*	**registrar el pulso**	*to take the pulse*
los cálculos	*stones*	**decidir**	*to decide*
los riñones	*kidneys*	**dentro de**	*within*

QUESTIONS ON READING

1. ¿Qué quiere saber la enfermera?
2. ¿Qué ha tenido el paciente?
3. ¿Cómo ha salido la operación?
4. ¿Qué hace la enfermera?
5. ¿Cómo está el paciente?
6. ¿Quién entra luego en el cuarto del paciente?
7. ¿Qué deciden la enfermera y el especialista?

Dialogue

PACIENTE: Doctor, he consultado con varios otros médicos pero necesito otra opinión. ¿Es necesaria la operación?

MÉDICO: Sí, señor. He pensado mucho en su caso y estoy de acuerdo con los otros médicos. La operación es necesaria y cuanto antes. Su condición ha empeorado.

PACIENTE: Pero doctor, no tengo mucho dinero. ¿Cómo voy a pagar los gastos del hospital?

MÉDICO: ¿No tiene Ud. seguro?

PACIENTE: No, no tengo seguro. No he trabajado en mucho tiempo.

MÉDICO: Entonces, Ud. tiene que recurrir a uno de los servicios sociales. En todo caso, tiene que pensar solamente en su estado de salud. Ud. está enfermo. Tenemos que operarle de los ojos. Tiene glaucoma.

PACIENTE: Sí, doctor, comprendo. Ya he sufrido mucho. Necesito la operación. Pero tengo mucho miedo.

MÉDICO: No debe tener miedo. El especialista que va a operarle tiene mucha experiencia en estos casos. Ud. no debe preocuparse.

PACIENTE: Bueno. Entonces voy a tratar de conseguir el dinero del Departamento de Seguro Social.

VOCABULARY

estar de acuerdo con   *to be in agreement with*
empeorar   *to get worse*
los gastos   *expenses, bills*
el seguro   *insurance*

recurrir a   *to have recourse to*
en todo caso   *in any case*
pensar en   *to think about*
el estado de salud   *state of health*
conseguir   *to get, obtain*

PATIENT: Doctor, I've consulted with several other doctors but I need another opinion. Is the operation necessary?

DOCTOR: Yes, sir. I have given a lot of thought to your case and I am in agreement with the other doctors. The operation is necessary and as soon as possible. Your condition has gotten worse.

PATIENT: But doctor, I don't have much money. How am I going to be able to pay the hospital bills?

DOCTOR: Don't you have insurance?

PATIENT: No, I don't have insurance. I haven't worked for a long time.

DOCTOR: Well then, you must seek the assistance of one of the social services. In any case, you must think only about your state of health. You are ill. We have to operate on your eyes. You have glaucoma.

PATIENT: Yes, doctor, I understand. I've already suffered a lot. I need the operation. But I'm very frightened.

DOCTOR: You shouldn't be afraid. The specialist who is going to operate on your eyes has a lot of experience in these cases. You shouldn't worry.

PATIENT: Very well. I'm going to try to get some money from the Department of Social Security.

QUESTIONS ON DIALOGUE

1. Según el médico, ¿es necesaria la operación?
2. ¿Tiene mucho dinero el señor? ¿Tiene seguro?
3. ¿A dónde puede recurrir el señor para recibir ayuda?
4. Según el médico, ¿en qué debe pensar solamente el señor?
5. ¿Cuál es la enfermedad que tiene el señor?
6. ¿Quién va a operarle al señor?
7. ¿Cómo va a conseguir el dinero el señor?

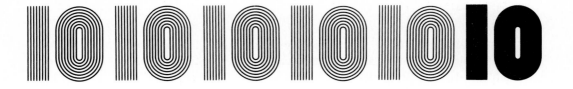

Grammar

COMMAND FORMS

The form that is used to give an order or to tell someone to do something is called the imperative or command form of the verb. For commands in English we simply use the basic form of the verb and omit the pronoun *you* (called "you understood"). Some examples of commands in English are *speak, run, stop.*

In Spanish, the command form for regular verbs is created simply by removing the ending of the infinitive and replacing it with what might be called the "opposite" letter or letters. That is, **-ar** is replaced with **-e** (for the singular **Ud.** form) or **-en** (for the plural **Uds.** form), and **-er** and **-ir** are both replaced by **-a** (for **Ud.**) or **-an** (for **Uds.**). For example:

hablar → **hable Ud.** or **hablen Uds.**
comer → **coma Ud.** or **coman Uds.**
escribir → **escriba Ud.** or **escriban Uds.**

To form a negative command, place the word **no** before the command form.

hable Ud. (*speak*) → **no hable Ud.** (*don't speak*)

When object pronouns and reflexive pronouns are involved, they *always* follow and are attached to the affirmative command form, but they must precede the negative command. When two object pronouns are used, the indirect pronoun always comes first.

Tome Ud. la medicina.	***Tóme*la* Ud.**	**No *la* tome Ud.**
Coma Ud. el pan.	**Cóma*lo* Ud.**	**No *lo* coma Ud.**
Escriba Ud. la carta.	**Escríba*la* Ud.**	**No *la* escriba Ud.**
Cómpreme la medicina.	***Cómpre*mela* Ud.**	**No *me la* compre Ud.**

* When one pronoun is attached to the command form, we must accentuate the form three syllables from the end; when two pronouns are attached to the command form, we must accentuate the form four syllables from the end.

The most common equivalent of the English *please* is **favor de,** which is combined with the infinitive to form an alternative to the direct command form. In addition to being more polite, it is also easier to use.

Hable Ud. despacio.	*Speak slowly.*
Favor de hablar despacio.	*Please speak slowly.*
Coma Ud. ahora.	*Eat now.*
Favor de comer ahora.	*Please eat now.*
Cómpreme la medicina.	*Buy me the medicine.*
Favor de comprarme la medicina.	*Please buy me the medicine.*

Oral practice

Change the following alternative command forms to direct commands.

Favor de hablar con el médico.	*Please speak with the doctor.*
Hable Ud. con el médico.	*Speak with the doctor.*

1. Favor de tomar las píldoras.
2. Favor de levantar los brazos.
3. Favor de caminar despacio.
4. Favor de doblar las rodillas.
5. Favor de descansar en cama.
6. Favor de esperar aquí.
7. Favor de trabajar.
8. Favor de consultar con el especialista.
9. Favor de beber el líquido.
10. Favor de responder a la pregunta.
11. Favor de leer la etiqueta.
12. Favor de comer más.
13. Favor de correr por aquí.
14. Favor de escribir su nombre.
15. Favor de abrir la boca.

Replace the direct object nouns with pronouns and put them in the appropriate place with respect to the verb.

Tomen Uds. las píldoras.	*Take the pills.*
Tómenlas Uds.	*Take them.*
No las tomen Uds.	*Don't take them.*

1. Compren Uds. las pastillas.
2. Beban Uds. el jarabe.
3. Levanten Uds. los brazos.
4. Cambien Uds. las camas.
5. Doblen Uds. las rodillas.
6. Lean Uds. los periódicos.
7. Terminen Uds. los ejercicios.
8. Limpien Uds. los cuartos.
9. Fumen Uds. los cigarrillos.
10. Coman Uds. el pan.
11. Tomen Uds. el regalo.
12. Escriban Uds. la dirección.
13. Usen Uds. el ungüento.
14. Preparen Uds. las recetas.
15. Abran Uds. las botellas.

Written practice

Translate the commands into Spanish.

1. Read (*Uds.*) the labels on the bottles.
2. Raise (*Ud.*) your left arm.
3. Consult (*Uds.*) with the surgeon.
4. Take (*Ud.*) these pills.
5. Don't smoke (*Uds.*) so much.
6. Buy (*Uds.*) the medicine.
7. Breathe (*Uds.*) deeply.
8. Cough (*Ud.*).
9. Open (*Ud.*) your mouth.
10. Don't eat (*Uds.*) now.

Translate the commands into English.

1. Cómprenme Uds. las cápsulas.
2. Llene Ud. las recetas en esta farmacia.
3. Señáleme Ud. donde le duele.
4. Respire Ud. profundamente.
5. Cálmense Uds.
6. Firmen Uds. aquí.
7. Llame Ud. por teléfono.
8. Enséñeme Ud. donde le duele.
9. Trate Ud. de mover las piernas.
10. Pasen Uds.

Grammar

IRREGULAR COMMAND FORMS

		SINGULAR	PLURAL
acercarse	*to approach*	acérquese Ud.	acérquense Uds.
acostarse	*to go to bed*	acuéstese Ud.	acuéstense Uds.
aplicarse	*to apply*	aplíquese Ud.	aplíquense Uds.
buscar	*to look for*	busque Ud.	busquen Uds.
cerrar	*to close*	cierre Ud.	cierren Uds.
decir	*to say, to tell*	diga Ud.	digan Uds.
despertarse	*to wake up*	despiértese Ud.	despiértense Uds.
dormir	*to sleep*	duerma Ud.	duerman Uds.
estar	*to be*	esté Ud.	estén Uds.
hacer	*to do, to make*	haga Ud.	hagan Uds.
indicar	*to indicate*	indique Ud.	indiquen Uds.
ir	*to go*	vaya Ud.	vayan Uds.
llegar	*to arrive*	llegue Ud.	lleguen Uds.
mostrar	*to show*	muestre Ud.	muestren Uds.
mover	*to move*	mueva Ud.	muevan Uds.
pagar	*to pay*	pague Ud.	paguen Uds.
poner	*to put, to place*	ponga Ud.	pongan Uds.
sacar	*to remove, to take out*	saque Ud.	saquen Uds.
sentarse	*to sit down*	siéntese Ud.	siéntense Uds.
ser	*to be*	sea Ud.	sean Uds.
tener	*to have*	tenga Ud.	tengan Uds.
tragar	*to swallow*	trague Ud.	traguen Uds.
venir	*to come*	venga Ud.	vengan Uds.
volver	*to return*	vuelva Ud.	vuelvan Uds.

Oral practice

Change the following alternative command forms to direct commands.

1. Favor de indicar dónde le duele.
2. Favor de dormir ocho horas.
3. Favor de volver en dos semanas.
4. Favor de buscar a la enfermera.
5. Favor de ir a la clínica hoy.
6. Favor de mover los pies.
7. Favor de sacar la lengua.
8. Favor de ponerse de pie.
9. Favor de decir la verdad.
10. Favor de pagarme ahora.
11. Favor de salir temprano.
12. Favor de sentarse aquí.
13. Favor de despertarse a las siete.
14. Favor de acostarse temprano.
15. Favor de hacer los ejercicios.
16. Favor de llegar a tiempo.
17. Favor de cerrar la boca.
18. Favor de venir a las cuatro.
19. Favor de hacer un puño.
20. Favor de mostrarme dónde le duele.

Change the following negative commands to affirmative commands.

No me lo compre Ud.
Cómpremelo Ud.

Don't buy it for me.
Buy it for me.

1. No me lo diga Ud.
2. No me lo lea Ud.
3. No me lo lleve Ud.
4. No me lo enseñe Ud.
5. No me lo haga Ud.
6. No me lo escriba Ud.
7. No me lo venda Ud.
8. No me lo muestre Ud.
9. No me lo aplique Ud.
10. No me lo pague Ud.

VOCABULARY

acostarse boca arriba   *to lie face up*
acostarse boca abajo   *to lie face down*
acostarse sobre el lado derecho
   to lie on the right side
acostarse sobre el lado izquierdo
   to lie on the left side

doblar la cabeza hacia adelante
   to bend your head forward
doblar la cabeza hacia atrás   *to bend*
   your head backward
doblar la cabeza a la derecha
   to bend your head to the right
doblar la cabeza a la izquierda
   to bend your head to the left

subir a la mesa   *to get on the table*
subir en la balanza   *to get on the scale*
bajar de la mesa   *to get down from the*
   table
quitarse la ropa   *to take off one's*
   clothing
desnudarse   *to take off one's clothing*
ponerse la ropa   *to put on one's*
   clothing
ponerse de pie   *to stand up*

Written practice

Translate the commands into Spanish using the **Ud.** form.

1. Lie face up.
2. Bend your head forward, now backward.
3. Get up on the table.
4. Take off your clothes.
5. Put on your clothes.

Translate the commands into English.

1. Suba en la balanza.
2. Acuéstese boca abajo.
3. Doble la cabeza a la derecha.
4. Desnúdese.
5. Póngase de pie.

Conversations

A: ¿Dónde le duele, señor?

B: Me duele la garganta.

A: Siéntese y quítese la camisa, por favor. Ahora, respire profundamente. ¿Tiene Ud. tos?

B: Sí, doctor. Hace tres días que tengo tos.

A: Abra la boca, por favor. Saque la lengua. Cierre la boca.

B: ¿Qué me pasa, doctor?

A: Ud. tiene un virus. Ud. necesita un antibiótico. Ahora, póngase la camisa. Ud. tiene que descansar mucho en cama.

A: Where does it hurt?

B: My throat hurts.

A: Sit down and take off your shirt, please. Now, breathe deeply. Do you have a cough?

B: Yes, doctor. I've had a cough for three days.

A: Open your mouth, please. Stick out your tongue. Close your mouth.

B: What's the matter with me, doctor?

A: You have a virus. You need an antibiotic. Now, put on your shirt. You must get a lot of bed rest.

A: No me siento bien, doctor.

B: Quítese la camisa y acuéstese boca arriba, por favor.

A: Tengo dolor en las articulaciones.

B: Doble la rodilla derecha, por favor. ¿Le duele mucho ahora?

A: Sí, doctor. Y me duele la espalda también.

B: Acuéstese boca abajo, ahora. ¿Le duele cuando le toco aquí?

A: I don't feel well, doctor.

B: Take off your shirt and lie face up, please.

A: I have pain in my joints.

B: Bend your right knee, please. Does it hurt a lot now?

A: Yes, doctor. And my back hurts also.

B: Lie face down, now. Does it hurt when I touch you here?

A: No, doctor.
B: Levante los brazos. ¿Le duele ahora?
A: Sí, doctor, mucho.
B: Bueno. Levántese y póngase la camisa.

A: Doctor, me duele la espalda y el hombro también.
B: Quítese la camisa y acuéstese boca abajo. Doble la cabeza hacia la derecha. Ahora doble la cabeza hacia la izquierda. Levante el brazo derecho.
A: ¿Qué debo hacer, doctor?
B: Ud. tiene una lesión de los músculos y debe descansar mucho.
A: No puedo porque tengo que trabajar.
B: Entonces, aplíquese este ungüento y tome estas píldoras para el dolor. Llámeme en dos semanas.

A: No, doctor.
B: Raise your arms. Does it hurt now?
A: Yes, doctor, a lot.
B: Very well. Get up and put on your shirt.

A: Doctor, my back hurts and also my shoulder.
B: Take off your shirt and lie face down. Bend your head toward the right. Now bend your head toward the left. Raise your right arm.
A: What should I do, doctor?
B: You have injured your muscles and you must get a lot of rest.
A: I can't because I have to work.
B: Well then, apply this ointment and take these pills for the pain. Call me in two weeks.

Vocabulary

PHYSICAL THERAPY/LA TERAPIA FÍSICA (LA FISIOTERAPIA)

la almohadilla eléctrica *electric heating pad*
las aplicaciones calientes *hot compresses*
bajarse de *to get off of, to go down*
el bastón *cane*
el (dedo) pulgar *thumb*
el (dedo) índice *index finger*
el (dedo) medio *middle finger*
el (dedo) anular *ring finger*
el (dedo) meñique *little finger*
los dedos de los pies *toes*
dejarle a uno *to let*
empujar *push*
la escalera *stairs, ladder*
hacer los ejercicios *to exercise*
hacer un puño *to make a fist*
la mano *hand*
la máquina *machine*
el aparato *machine*

la máquina ultrasónica *ultrasound machine*
el masaje *massage*
las muletas *crutches*
el parálisis *paralysis*
poner en cabestrillo *to put in a sling*
poner en yeso *to put in a cast*
enyesar *to put in a cast*
la silla de ruedas *wheelchair*
el soporte *brace*
subir a *to go up, to get on*
el (la) terapeuta *therapist*
el (la) terapista *therapist*
el torniquete *tourniquet*
los tratamientos *treatments*
tratar de mover los pies, los brazos, etc. *to try to move your feet, arms, etc.*

Oral practice

Answer the questions using the cues.

¿Qué trata de mover el paciente?   *What is the patient trying to move?*
El paciente trata de mover el dedo.   *The patient is trying to move his finger.*

1. ¿Qué trata de mover el niño?   • right leg
2. ¿Qué trata de mover la muchacha?   • left arm
3. ¿Qué trata de mover el hombre?   • right arm
4. ¿Qué trata de mover la joven?   • legs
5. ¿Qué trata de mover la mujer?   • arms
6. ¿Qué puede mover la paciente?   • head
7. ¿Qué puede mover la niña?   • little finger
8. ¿Qué puede mover el joven?   • thumb
9. ¿Qué puede mover el anciano?   • feet
10. ¿Qué puede mover el muchacho?   • toes

Answer the questions with complete sentences.

1. ¿Es Ud. el terapista físico?
2. ¿Puede Ud. ayudarme a hacer los ejercicios?
3. ¿Puede Ud. enseñarme a manejar las muletas?
4. ¿Hace los ejercicios el hombre?
5. ¿Quiere Ud. descansar un rato?
6. ¿Necesita Ud. descansar?
7. ¿Puede Ud. mover las piernas?
8. ¿Le duele cuando le toco aquí?
9. ¿Puede Ud. mover los dedos de los pies?
10. ¿Sabe Ud. usar la máquina ultrasónica?

Change the following alternative command forms to direct commands.

1. Favor de empujar.
2. Favor de hacer un puño.
3. Favor de hacer los ejercicios.
4. Favor de subir la escalera.
5. Favor de bajar la escalera.
6. Favor de usar un bastón.
7. Favor de mover el dedo meñique.
8. Favor de mover los pies.
9. Favor de mover los dedos.
10. Favor de mover el brazo izquierdo.
11. Favor de acercarse a la máquina.
12. Favor de ponerse de pie.
13. Favor de mover el dedo pulgar (el pulgar).
14. Favor de usar las muletas.
15. Favor de sentarse.

Dialogue

TERAPISTA: Buenos días, señor Gómez. ¿Cómo se siente Ud. hoy?
PACIENTE: Me siento mucho mejor, gracias. Pero todavía me duele la muñeca.
TERAPISTA: Sí, por supuesto. Sólo hace una semana que viene aquí. Debe venir por seis meses para curarse del todo.
PACIENTE: ¿Por qué tengo que hacer tantas visitas?
TERAPISTA: Ud. se ha fracturado la muñeca y estos ejercicios son muy graduales. Ahora, agárrese de la barra y tire.
PACIENTE: Eso me duele.
TERAPISTA: No tire tan fuertemente. Ahora, haga un puño.
PACIENTE: Eso es un poco más fácil.
TERAPISTA: Ahora, mueva los dedos, uno a uno. Primero el pulgar, entonces el índice, y luego el meñique.
PACIENTE: Eso es muy difícil.
TERAPISTA: Sí, pero este ejercicio es muy importante, y dentro de poco, va a ser mucho más fácil.
PACIENTE: Espero que sí.
TERAPISTA: Sí, sin duda. Eso es todo por hoy. No se olvide de la próxima cita, el martes a las dos y media. Trate de hacer los ejercicios en casa.
PACIENTE: Muchas gracias, señorita. Hasta la próxima cita.

VOCABULARY

todavía   *still*
por supuesto   *of course*
curarse   *to become cured, get better*
fracturar   *to break, fracture*
agarrarse de   *to grab, hold on to*
las barras paralelas   *parallel bars*
tirar   *to pull*

THERAPIST: Good morning, Mr. Gómez. How do you feel today?
PATIENT: I feel much better, thank you. But my wrist still hurts.
THERAPIST: Yes, of course. You have only been coming here for a week. You must come for six months in order to be completely cured.
PATIENT: Why do I have to make so many visits?
THERAPIST: You've fractured your wrist and these exercises are done gradually. Now, grab on to the bar and pull.
PATIENT: That hurts.
THERAPIST: Don't pull so forcefully. Now, make a fist.
PATIENT: That's a little easier.
THERAPIST: Now, move your fingers, one by one. First, the thumb, then the index finger, and next the little one.
PATIENT: That's very difficult.

THERAPIST: Yes, but this exercise is very important, and in a little while it will be much easier.

PATIENT: I hope so.

THERAPIST: Yes, without a doubt. That's all for today. Don't forget the next appointment, Tuesday at two-thirty. Try to do the exercises at home.

PATIENT: Thanks a lot, miss. Until the next appointment.

QUESTIONS ON DIALOGUE

1. ¿Cómo se siente el señor Gómez?
2. ¿Qué le duele?
3. ¿Por qué tiene que hacer muchas visitas el señor?
4. ¿Qué ejercicios hace?
5. ¿Cuándo es su próxima cita con la terapista?

Vocabulary

MEDICINES/LAS MEDICINAS

el agua mineral *mineral water*
los analgésicos *analgesics*
los antibióticos *antibiotics*
las antihistaminas *antihistamines*
los calmantes *sedatives*
el jarabe para la tos *cough syrup*

la leche de magnesia *milk of magnesia*
el linimento *liniment*
los sedantes *sedatives*
los tranquilizantes *tranquilizers*

Grammar

PRESENT INDICATIVE OF THE IRREGULAR VERB *DAR* (TO GIVE)

yo	**doy**	*I give*
él/ella	**da**	*he/she gives*
Ud.	**da**	*you give*
nosotros/nosotras	**damos**	*we give*
ellos/ellas	**dan**	*they give*
Uds.	**dan**	*you* (pl.) *give*

Oral practice

Change the sentences using the cues.

1. La enfermera les da los tranquilizantes a los pacientes.
   - los enfermeros   • el médico y yo   • el asistente   • yo

2. El enfermero les da el jarabe a los pacientes.
   ● nosotros   ● los médicos   ● las enfermeras   ● la asistenta

3. El farmacéutico le da la leche de magnesia a mi madre.
   ● yo   ● mi padre   ● nosotros   ● mi hermana

Answer the questions with complete sentences.

1. ¿Quién está dando la medicina a la paciente?
2. ¿Quién está dando los analgésicos al hombre?
3. ¿Quién está dando la leche de magnesia a la muchacha?
4. ¿Quién está dando el antibiótico al paciente?
5. ¿Quién está dando los calmantes a los pacientes?

VOCABULARY

necesitar *to need to*
es necesario *it is necessary to*
antes de comer *before eating*
después de comer *after eating*
antes de acostarse *before bedtime*

al despertarse *upon awakening*
una vez al día *once a day*
dos veces al día *twice a day*
cada seis horas *every six hours*
según la etiqueta *according to the label*

Answer the questions with complete sentences.

1. ¿Es necesario darme la medicina ahora?
2. ¿Es necesario darle el antibiótico al paciente?
3. ¿A qué hora tiene Ud. que dar la medicina a la mujer?
4. ¿Tengo que tomar la píldora antes de acostarme?
5. ¿Necesito usar el ungüento al despertarme?
6. ¿Me aplico el linimento dos veces al día?
7. ¿Es necesario tomar el antibiótico cada seis horas?
8. ¿Debo tomar la medicina antes de comer?
9. ¿Necesita la mujer tomar el analgésico ahora?
10. ¿Debe Ud. dar el tranquilizante a la madre ahora?

Answer the questions using the cues.

¿Cuándo debo tomar la medicina?   *When should I take the medicine?*
Ud. debe tomar la medicina una vez al día.   *You should take the medicine once a day.*

1. ¿Cuándo debe tomar las píldoras mi madre?
2. ¿Cuándo tengo que tomar los antibióticos?
3. ¿Cuándo tiene que tomar el líquido el hombre?
4. ¿Cuándo necesita tomar las pastillas mi padre?
5. ¿Cuándo debe la muchacha tomar el jarabe para la tos?
6. ¿Cuándo debe tomar el tranquilizante mi hermana?
7. ¿Cuándo tiene que usar el linimento la mujer?

● when she awakens
● every six hours
● before eating
● four times a day
● according to the label
● right now
● before bedtime

8. ¿Cuándo necesito usar las gotas?
9. ¿Cuándo debo aplicarme el ungüento?
10. ¿Cuándo debo usar la leche de magnesia?

- every six hours
- upon awakening
- before going to bed

Answer the questions with complete sentences.

1. ¿Quién le ha dado la medicina a Ud.?
2. ¿Le ha dado Ud. la receta al farmacéutico?
3. ¿Les han dado las enfermeras los analgésicos a los pacientes?
4. ¿Le ha dado la enfermera el jarabe al paciente?
5. ¿Les han dado Uds. las píldoras a las pacientes?

Conversations

A: ¿Qué me da para mi mal, doctor?

B: Le doy estas cápsulas.
A: ¿Cuántas veces al día tomo las cápsulas?
B: Debe tomarlas tres veces al día, una hora antes de comer.

A: ¿Me receta algo, doctor?

B: Sí, le receto un antibiótico.

A: ¿Cuántas veces al día tomo los antibióticos?
B: Debe tomarlos cada seis horas, antes de comer.

A: ¿Me da algo para el dolor, doctor?

B: Sí, le doy este ungüento.
A: ¿Cuándo tengo que aplicármelo?
B: Tres veces al día.

A: ¿Qué me da para la tos, doctor?

B: Le doy un jarabe.
A: ¿Cuántas veces al día debo tomarlo?

B: Debe tomar una cucharada cada cuatro horas, y siempre antes de acostarse.

A: What are you giving me for my illness, doctor?

B: I'm giving you these capsules.
A: How many times a day do I take the capsules?
B: You must take them three times a day, one hour before eating.

A: Are you prescribing something for me, doctor?

B: Yes, I'm prescribing an antibiotic for you.

A: How many times a day do I take the antibiotics?
B: You should take them every six hours, before eating.

A: Are you giving me something for the pain, doctor?

B: Yes, I'm giving you this ointment.
A: When do I have to apply it?
B: Three times a day.

A: What are you giving me for my cough, doctor?

B: I'm giving you this syrup.
A: How many times a day should I take it?

B: You should take a tablespoonful every four hours, and always before bedtime.

A: ¿Qué me da para la nariz tupida, doctor?

A: What are you giving me for my stuffy nose, doctor?

B: Le doy estas gotas.

B: I'm giving you these drops.

A: ¿Cuándo tengo que tomar las gotas?

A: When must I take the drops?

B: Tiene que tomarlas cada seis horas.

B: You must take them every six hours.

A: ¿Qué puedo tomar para el estreñimiento, doctor?

A: What can I take for my constipation, doctor?

B: Debe tomar la leche de magnesia.

B: You should take milk of magnesia.

A: ¿Cuándo debo tomar la leche de magnesia?

A: When should I take the milk of magnesia?

B: Debe tomar dos cucharadas tres veces al día.

B: You should take two tablespoonfuls three times a day.

Grammar

PRESENT INDICATIVE OF THE IRREGULAR VERB *PONER* (TO PUT, TO PLACE, TO GIVE)

yo	**pongo**	*I put*
él/ella	**pone**	*he/she puts*
Ud.	**pone**	*you put*
nosotros/nosotras	**ponemos**	*we put*
ellos/ellas	**ponen**	*they put*
Uds.	**ponen**	*you* (pl.) *put*

This verb usually means *to put* or *to place,* as in the following examples:

Pongo las flores en el cuarto del paciente.

I'm putting the flowers in the patient's room.

Ponemos los libros en la mesa.

We're putting the books on the table.

This verb means *to give* when we refer to injections, as in these examples:

El médico me va a poner una inyección de penicilina.

The doctor is going to give me a penicillin injection.

Le pongo a Ud. una inyección de antibiótico.

I'm giving you an injection of antibiotic.

When **poner** is used reflexively with a noun it means *to put on* or *to wear,* as in:

Me pongo la camisa.

I'm putting on my shirt.

La paciente se pone la blusa.

The patient is putting on her blouse.

When **poner** is used reflexively with an adjective it means *to become,* as in these examples:

La mujer se pone nerviosa.	*The woman is becoming nervous.*
El hombre se pone triste.	*The man is becoming sad.*

VOCABULARY

la diabetis   *diabetes*
el coma diabético   *diabetic coma*
la inmunización   *immunization*
inmunizar   *immunize*
la influenza   *flu*
inocular   *innoculate*
la inyección de antibiótico   *antibiotic injection*

la inyección de insulina   *insulin injection*
la inyección de penicilina   *penicillin injection*
la inyección de refuerzo   *booster shot*
la inyección intravenosa   *intravenous injection*
inyectar   *inject*
la vacuna   *vaccine*

Oral practice

Change the sentences using the cues.

1. El médico le pone la inyección a la paciente.
   - la doctora   • yo   • el cirujano   • el anestesiólogo

2. La enfermera les pone unas vacunas para las paperas a las niñas.
   - las enfermeras   • los médicos   • el médico   • el médico y yo

3. Las asistentas les ponen unas vacunas para la influenza a los hombres.
   - nosotros   • la enfermera y yo   • la enfermera   • los enfermeros

Answer the questions with complete sentences.

1. ¿Les pone Ud. unas vacunas para la influenza a los hombres?
2. ¿Les ponen los médicos unas vacunas para la rubéola a los niños?
3. ¿Les pone el médico unas vacunas para la poliomielitis a sus hijos?
4. ¿Le pone la enfermera una vacuna para el tétano al joven?
5. ¿Le pone Ud. una vacuna para la difteria al paciente?

Answer the questions by following the model.

¿Le ha puesto el médico la inyección de penicilina?	*Has the doctor given you the penicillin injection?*
Sí, el médico me ha puesto la inyección de penicilina.	*Yes, the doctor has given me the penicillin injection.*

1. ¿Les han puesto las enfermeras las inyecciones intravenosas a los pacientes?
2. ¿Le ha puesto la doctora la vacuna para la tos ferina al muchacho?

3. ¿Les han puesto los médicos las inyecciones de antibiótico a los hombres?
4. ¿Les han puesto Uds. las vacunas para la escarlatina a los niños?
5. ¿Le ha puesto Ud. la vacuna para la malaria a la mujer?

Answer the questions with complete sentences.

1. ¿Es necesario ponerles las vacunas a los niños?
2. ¿Necesita mi hija una inyección de refuerzo?
3. ¿Tiene Ud. que inocular a mi hijo?
4. ¿Tiene Ud. que ponerles las inyecciones a los pacientes?
5. ¿Necesita Ud. inmunizar a los pacientes?

Written practice

Translate the sentences into Spanish.

1. The doctor has already given her the penicillin injection.
2. The nurse has to give me the injection.
3. He is putting on his shirt now.
4. She has put the flowers in her room.
5. You must take the medicine before you go to bed.
6. Who gave him the pills?
7. You shouldn't take so many tranquilizers.
8. I'm giving you an injection of antibiotic.
9. Where have you put the books?
10. She is getting very nervous.

Conversations

A: ¿Qué me va a poner, doctor?

B: Le pongo una inyección para el catarro.

A: ¿Qué puedo tomar para el catarro?

B: Tiene que tomar estas cápsulas.

A: ¿Cuántas veces al día debo tomar las cápsulas?

B: Ud. tiene que tomarlas cada cuatro horas.

A: ¿Está enferma su hermana?

B: Tiene diabetis.

A: ¿Qué tiene que hacer para la diabetis?

A: What are you going to give me, doctor?

B: I'm giving you an injection for your cold.

A: What can I take for my cold?

B: You have to take these capsules.

A: How many times a day should I take the capsules?

B: You must take them every four hours.

A: Is your sister sick?

B: She has diabetes.

A: What does she have to do for the diabetes?

B: Tiene que ponerse las inyecciones de insulina.

A: ¿Qué más tiene que hacer?

B: Tiene que seguir una dieta especial.

B: She has to give herself insulin injections.

A: What else does she have to do?

B: She has to follow a special diet.

Grammar

THE FUTURE TENSE

The future tense of regular verbs is formed by adding the personal endings to the infinitive (not just the stem). The personal endings are the same for the **-ar, -er,** and **-ir** verbs. In English the future is expressed by using the auxiliary verbs *will* or *shall.*

yo	**hablaré**	*I will speak*
él/ella	**hablará**	*he/she will speak*
Ud.	**hablará**	*you will speak*
nosotros/nosotras	**hablaremos**	*we will speak*
ellos/ellas	**hablarán**	*they will speak*
Uds.	**hablarán**	*you (pl.) will speak*

Oral practice

Change the sentences to the future tense following the model.

El médico come en casa ahora.
El médico comerá en casa más tarde.

The doctor is eating at home now.
The doctor will eat at home later.

1. El hombre toma los analgésicos ahora.
2. Compramos las antihistaminas ahora.
3. Me aplico el linimento ahora.
4. Uso el ungüento ahora.
5. Mi madre consulta con el especialista ahora.
6. El médico me receta las píldoras ahora.
7. Lleno la receta ahora.
8. La enfermera le da el jarabe al paciente ahora.
9. El farmacéutico prepara la receta ahora.
10. Mi abuelo necesita el agua mineral ahora.
11. Bebo la leche de magnesia ahora.
12. Comemos ahora.
13. Voy a la farmacia ahora.
14. Escribo la carta ahora.
15. Las enfermeras abren las ventanas ahora.

Answer the questions with complete sentences.

1. ¿A qué hora tomará Ud. la medicina?
2. ¿Cuándo consultará la madre con el pediatra?
3. ¿Dónde comprarán Uds. los tranquilizantes?
4. ¿Quién recetará los antibióticos?
5. ¿Cuándo comerán los pacientes?
6. ¿Beberán los hombres el jarabe?
7. ¿Correrán Uds. mucho?
8. ¿Dónde vivirán sus padres?
9. ¿Quién escribirá las cartas?
10. ¿Quién irá con la doctora?

Grammar

FUTURE TENSE OF IRREGULAR VERBS

decir	diré	dirá	dirá	diremos	dirán	dirán
haber	habré	habrá	habrá	habremos	habrán	habrán
hacer	haré	hará	hará	haremos	harán	harán
poder	podré	podrá	podrá	podremos	podrán	podrán
poner	pondré	pondrá	pondrá	pondremos	pondrán	pondrán
querer	querré	querrá	querrá	querremos	querrán	querrán
saber	sabré	sabrá	sabrá	sabremos	sabrán	sabrán
salir	saldré	saldrá	saldrá	saldremos	saldrán	saldrán
tener	tendré	tendrá	tendrá	tendremos	tendrán	tendrán
venir	vendré	vendrá	vendrá	vendremos	vendrán	vendrán

Oral practice

Change the sentences to the future tense following the model.

Su padre viene hoy. *His father is coming today.*
Su padre vendrá pasado mañana. *His father will come the day after tomorrow.*

1. El enfermero me pone la inyección hoy.
2. El paciente sale del hospital hoy.
3. Tengo que ir a la clínica hoy.
4. El técnico hace el análisis hoy.
5. Hacemos los ejercicios hoy.
6. La paciente puede caminar hoy.

7. Los médicos tienen los resultados hoy.
8. La paciente quiere salir del hospital hoy.
9. Las doctoras hacen los exámenes hoy.
10. Los técnicos hacen las radiografías hoy.

Answer the questions with complete sentences.

1. ¿Tendré que volver al hospital?
2. ¿Me hará el examen la doctora?
3. ¿Vendrán a visitarme sus padres?
4. ¿Me dirán la verdad los médicos?
5. ¿Harán Uds. los ejercicios en casa?

Conversations

A: ¿Cuándo tendrá el médico los resultados de las pruebas?

A: When will the doctor have the results of the tests?

B: Dice que los recibirá en unos días.

B: He says that he'll receive them in a few days.

A: ¿Le van a operar a Ud.?

A: Are they going to operate on you?

B: Depende de los resultados.

B: It depends on the results.

A: ¿Qué dice su marido?

A: What does your husband say?

B: Dice que no les permitirá operar.

B: He says that he won't permit them to operate.

A: ¿Cuándo podré salir del hospital?

A: When will I be able to leave the hospital?

B: La doctora le examinará esta tarde y le dirá cuándo podrá salir.

B: The doctor will examine you this afternoon and she'll tell you when you'll be able to leave.

A: ¿Debo seguir tomando el medicamento en casa?

A: Must I still use the medication at home?

B: Sí, y tendrá que seguir la dieta también.

B: Yes, and you will have to follow the diet also.

A: ¿Recuperaré pronto si sigo la dieta?

A: Will I recuperate soon if I follow the diet?

B: Sí, sin duda. Ud. recuperará pronto.

B: Yes, without a doubt, you will recuperate soon.

Written practice

Translate the sentences into Spanish.

1. The nurse has given the medication to the patient.
2. When will he have to take the pills?
3. Will you prescribe an antibiotic for her?

4. Take this medicine every four hours.
5. He has applied the ointment on his arm.
6. She has to give the injections to the patients.
7. You must go to the doctor for your flu injection.
8. When will the doctor receive the results of the tests?
9. Will she have to stay in the hospital for a long time?
10. Is it necessary to give him an injection now?

Dialogue

ENFERMERA: Buenas tardes, señora. ¿Cuál es su problema?

SEÑORA: Buenas tardes, señorita. Los oficiales de la escuela me han dicho que mis hijos no podrán asistir porque no les han puesto unas vacunas.

ENFERMERA: Eso es cierto.

SEÑORA: ¿Les ponen las vacunas aquí, en la clínica?

ENFERMERA: Sí, es uno de los servicios que ofrecemos.

SEÑORA: ¿Me costará mucho dinero?

ENFERMERA: No, señora. Es un servicio gratuito. ¿Cuántos hijos tiene Ud.?

SEÑORA: Tengo dos hijos y una hija.

ENFERMERA: ¿Cuántos años tienen?

SEÑORA: El mayor tiene doce años, la niña tiene diez, y el menor tiene siete años.

ENFERMERA: Muy bien. Tenemos que ponerles una vacuna para el sarampión y una vacuna para la viruela. Además, debemos hacerles una prueba de tuberculosis.

SEÑORA: Esas son muchas vacunas.

ENFERMERA: Sí, pero son muy importantes para la salud de sus hijos.

SEÑORA: ¿Quién les pondrá las vacunas?

ENFERMERA: El médico se encargará de eso. ¿Están aquí ahora sus hijos?

SEÑORA: Sí, están en la sala de espera.

ENFERMERA: Bien. Ud. puede traerlos al consultorio y el médico les pondrá las vacunas en unos minutos.

SEÑORA: Muchas gracias, señorita.

ENFERMERA: De nada, señora.

VOCABULARY

los oficiales *officials*
la escuela *school*
el servicio *service*
ofrecer *to offer*
costar *to cost*
gratuito *free*
el (la) mayor *the older one, the oldest*
el (la) menor *the younger one, the youngest*

el sarampión *measles*
la viruela *smallpox*
la prueba de tuberculosis *tuberculosis test*
la salud *health*
encargarse de *to take care of, to take over*
la sala de espera *waiting room*
de nada *you're welcome*

NURSE: Good afternoon, ma'am. What is your problem?

WOMAN: Good afternoon, miss. The school officials have told me that my children will not be able to attend school because they haven't been given some vaccines.

NURSE: That's true.

WOMAN: Do they give vaccines here in the clinic?

NURSE: Yes, it's one of the services that we offer.

WOMAN: Will it cost me a lot of money?

NURSE: No, ma'am. It's a free service. How many children do you have?

WOMAN: I have two sons and a daughter.

NURSE: How old are they?

WOMAN: The older boy is twelve years old, the girl is ten, and the youngest is seven.

NURSE: Very well. We have to give them a vaccine for measles and a vaccine for smallpox. In addition, we must do a tuberculosis test.

WOMAN: Those are a lot of vaccines.

NURSE: Yes, but they are important for your children's health.

WOMAN: Who is going to give them the vaccines?

NURSE: The doctor will take care of that. Are your children here now?

WOMAN: Yes, they're in the waiting room.

NURSE: Good. You can bring them to the office and the doctor will give them the vaccines in a few minutes.

WOMAN: Thank you very much, miss.

NURSE: You're welcome, ma'am.

QUESTIONS ON DIALOGUE

1. ¿Por qué no podrán asistir a la escuela los hijos de la señora?
2. ¿Les pondrán las vacunas en la clínica?
3. ¿Costarán mucho dinero las vacunas?
4. ¿Cuántos hijos tiene la señora?
5. ¿Cuántos años tienen sus hijos?
6. ¿Contra qué enfermedades deben ponerles las vacunas?
7. ¿Deben hacerles una prueba de tuberculosis?
8. ¿Para qué son importantes las vacunas?
9. ¿Quién les pondrá las vacunas?
10. ¿Cuándo les pondrá las vacunas?

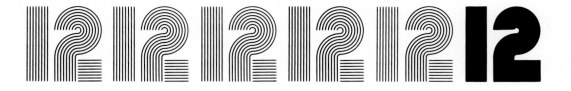

Grammar

PRETERITE TENSE OF THE FIRST CONJUGATION

yo	**hablé**	*I spoke*
él/ella	**habló**	*he/she spoke*
Ud.	**habló**	*you spoke*
nosotros/nosotras	**hablamos**	*we spoke*
ellos/ellas	**hablaron**	*they spoke*
Uds.	**hablaron**	*you* (pl.) *spoke*

Spanish has two simple tenses to express things that have occurred in the past. The preterite tense is used to indicate a completed past action. For example:

Mi madre se cortó con un cuchillo ayer.	*My mother cut herself with a knife yesterday.*
Yo le llamé al médico a las tres.	*I called the doctor at three.*
El hombre compró la medicina anteanoche.	*The man bought the medicine the night before last.*
Entramos en el cuarto de la paciente.	*We entered the patient's room.*
Mi hermana llenó todos los formularios.	*My sister filled out all the forms.*

It is also used to indicate an action which occurred within a specific time period.

Yo hablé con el médico por dos horas.	*I spoke with the doctor for two hours.*
Ella consultó con el especialista por una hora.	*She consulted with the specialist for an hour.*

It is also used with the verb form **hace** plus a specific time period to express the English *ago*. Look at the following examples:

¿Cuánto tiempo hace que visitó Ud. a sus tíos?
How long ago did you visit your aunt and uncle?

Hace dos meses que los visité.
I visited them two months ago.

Oral practice

Answer the questions in the preterite tense following the model.

¿Habló Ud. con el especialista?
Did you speak with the specialist?

Sí, hablé con el especialista.
Yes, I spoke with the specialist.

1. ¿Tomó Ud. las píldoras?
2. ¿Llamó Ud. a la enfermera?
3. ¿Entró Ud. en el cuarto?
4. ¿Estudió Ud. la medicina?
5. ¿Recetó Ud. las píldoras?
6. ¿Trabajó Ud. en la clínica?
7. ¿Consultó Ud. con el médico?
8. ¿Dobló Ud. la pierna derecha?
9. ¿Aceptó Ud. la decisión del médico?
10. ¿Usó Ud. el linimento?

Change from the singular to the plural.

Consulté con el especialista ayer.
I consulted with the specialist yesterday.

Consultamos con el especialista ayer.
We consulted with the specialist yesterday.

1. El niño tomó la medicina anoche.
2. La madre consultó con el especialista ayer.
3. El especialista me llamó anoche.
4. El cirujano me amputó la pierna ayer.
5. La enfermera calmó al paciente esta mañana.
6. La mujer limpió los cuartos anoche.
7. La doctora visitó a la paciente a las tres de la tarde.
8. El cirujano operó esta mañana.
9. Llené las recetas anteayer.
10. El joven compró la medicina a las ocho de la mañana.

Grammar

PRETERITE TENSE OF THE SECOND CONJUGATION

yo	**comí**	*I ate*
él/ella	**comió**	*he/she ate*
Ud.	**comió**	*you ate*
nosotros/nosotras	**comimos**	*we ate*
ellos/ellas	**comieron**	*they ate*
Uds.	**comieron**	*you (pl.) ate*

Oral practice

Answer the questions in the preterite tense following the model.

¿Comió Ud. tarde?   *Did you eat late?*
Sí, comí tarde.   *Yes, I ate late.*

1. ¿Bebió Ud. la leche?
2. ¿Vendió Ud. la medicina?
3. ¿Corrió Ud. mucho?
4. ¿Aprendió Ud. a hablar inglés?
5. ¿Comprendió Ud. la lección?
6. ¿Volvió Ud. a la clínica?
7. ¿Respondió Ud. a las preguntas?
8. ¿Comprendió Ud. la situación?
9. ¿Comió Ud. temprano?
10. ¿Volvió Ud. al hospital?

Answer the questions in the preterite tense following the model.

¿Volvieron Uds. al hospital?   *Did you return to the hospital?*
Sí, volvimos al hospital.   *Yes, we returned to the hospital.*

1. ¿Respondieron Uds. a las preguntas de la recepcionista?
2. ¿Comieron Uds. temprano?
3. ¿Vendieron Uds. la medicina?
4. ¿Bebieron Uds. el jugo?
5. ¿Corrieron Uds. por el parque?
6. ¿Aprendieron Uds. a hablar español?
7. ¿Vendieron Uds. la casa?
8. ¿Comieron Uds. tarde?
9. ¿Comprendieron Uds. la explicación del médico?
10. ¿Volvieron Uds. al laboratorio?

Grammar

PRETERITE TENSE OF THE THIRD CONJUGATION

yo	**abrí**	*I opened*
él/ella	**abrió**	*he/she opened*
Ud.	**abrió**	*you opened*
nosotros/nosotras	**abrimos**	*we opened*
ellos/ellas	**abrieron**	*they opened*
Uds.	**abrieron**	*you (pl.) opened*

Oral practice

Answer the questions in the preterite tense following the model.

¿Abrió Ud. las ventanas?   *Did you open the windows?*
Sí, abrí las ventanas.   *Yes, I opened the windows.*

1. ¿Salió Ud. tarde?
2. ¿Decidió Ud. ir al hospital?
3. ¿Recibió Ud. los resultados de las pruebas?
4. ¿Sufrió Ud. mucho después de la operación?
5. ¿Recibió Ud. el dinero?
6. ¿Vivió Ud. cerca del hospital?
7. ¿Escribió Ud. las cartas?
8. ¿Recibió Ud. las píldoras?
9. ¿Escribió Ud. la receta?
10. ¿Recibió Ud. el dinero?

Change the sentences using the cues.

1. El paciente recibió el regalo ayer.
2. Decidimos volver al hospital ayer.
3. Escribí las listas ayer.
4. La mujer salió de la clínica ayer.
5. Los hombres recibieron el dinero ayer.

- last month
- the night before last
- last week
- this morning
- this afternoon

Vocabulary

EMERGENCY SITUATIONS/CASOS DE EMERGENCIA

el accidente   *accident*
ahogarse   *to drown, suffocate, choke, smother*
la ambulancia   *ambulance*
el antídoto   *antidote*
apuñalar   *to stab*
atacar   *to attack*
el ataque al corazón   *heart attack*
atentar el suicidio   *to attempt to commit suicide*
la camilla   *stretcher*
el camillero   *stretcher bearer*
el cuchillo   *knife*
desmayarse   *to faint*
la dosis excesiva   *overdose*
las drogas   *drugs*
envenenarse   *to poison oneself*
escupir sangre   *to spit up blood*
estar sangrando   *to bleed*
fracturar, romper   *to fracture, break*
hacerse daño, lesionarse   *to hurt oneself*

la hemorragia   *hemorrhage*
la herida   *wound*
hospitalizar   *to hospitalize*
llevar en camilla   *to carry on a stretcher*
masticar   *to chew*
ocurrir   *to occur*
el oxígeno   *oxygen*
perder el conocimiento   *to lose consciousness*
la pistola   *pistol*
poner en yeso   *to put in a cast*
enyesar   *to put in a cast*
los puntos   *stitches*
la quemadura   *burn*
quemarse   *to burn oneself*
la respiración artificial   *artificial respiration*
la respiración artificial boca a boca   *mouth-to-mouth resuscitation*
el revólver   *revolver*

la sala de cuidado intensivo
  intensive care unit
la sala de emergencia   *emergency room*
tocar   *to touch*

tragar   *to swallow*
la venda   *bandage*
el vendaje   *bandage, dressing*
vendar   *to bandage*
el veneno   *poison*

Oral practice

Answer the questions with complete sentences in the preterite.

1. ¿Quién se cortó con un cuchillo?
2. ¿Llevaron al hombre en camilla?
3. ¿Se fracturó el brazo el joven?
4. ¿Atentó el suicidio el hombre?
5. ¿Se ahogó el niño?
6. ¿Lo apuñaló Ud. a su cuñado?
7. ¿Se desmayó la mujer?
8. ¿Cuándo se lesionó Ud.?
9. ¿Se envenenó la joven?
10. ¿Hospitalizaron a la muchacha?

Written practice

Translate the sentences into Spanish.

1. Where did the accident occur?
2. Why did he take the poison?
3. Why did the young girl try to commit suicide?
4. He stabbed the man three times.
5. The child spit up blood.
6. They sent an ambulance.
7. What happened to you?
8. They put the arm in a cast.
9. The doctor gave me ten stitches.
10. He lost consciousness.

Conversations

A: ¿Qué le pasó al niño?
B: Su madre lo dejó solo en casa y se quemó.
A: ¿Cómo se quemó?
B: Encendió unos fósforos en la cocina.
A: ¿Es grave su condición?
B: Sí, está en la sala de cuidado intensivo.

A: What happened to the child?
B: His mother left him alone at home and he got burned.
A: How did he burn himself?
B: He lit some matches in the kitchen.
A: Is his condition serious?
B: Yes, he's in the intensive care unit.

A: ¿Dónde ocurrió el accidente?
B: Ocurrió en la calle.
A: ¿Qué le pasó al hombre?

A: Where did the accident occur?
B: It occurred in the street.
A: What happened to the man?

B: Sufrió un ataque al corazón.
A: ¿Mandaron una ambulancia?
B: Sí, lo llevaron al hospital.
A: ¿Notificaron a su familia?
B: Sí, llamaron a su esposa.

B: He had a heart attack.
A: Did they send an ambulance?
B: Yes, they brought him to the hospital.
A: Did they notify his family?
B: Yes, they called his wife.

Grammar

PRETERITE TENSE OF IRREGULAR VERBS

These verbs are irregular only in the first person singular of the preterite tense.

aplicar	apliqué	aplicó	aplicó	aplicamos	aplicaron	aplicaron
atacar	ataqué	atacó	atacó	atacamos	atacaron	atacaron
buscar	busqué	buscó	buscó	buscamos	buscaron	buscaron
explicar	expliqué	explicó	explicó	explicamos	explicaron	explicaron
indicar	indiqué	indicó	indicó	indicamos	indicaron	indicaron
llegar	llegué	llegó	llegó	llegamos	llegaron	llegaron
masticar	mastiqué	masticó	masticó	masticamos	masticaron	masticaron
pagar	pagué	pagó	pagó	pagamos	pagaron	pagaron
sacar	saqué	sacó	sacó	sacamos	sacaron	sacaron
tocar	toqué	tocó	tocó	tocamos	tocaron	tocaron
tragar	tragué	tragó	tragó	tragamos	tragaron	tragaron

Oral practice

Answer the questions in the affirmative.

1. ¿Llegó Ud. tarde?
2. ¿Se aplicó Ud. el ungüento?
3. ¿Le explicó Ud. la situación a la mujer?
4. ¿Tragó Ud. el líquido?
5. ¿Masticó Ud. las pastillas?
6. ¿Pagó Ud. en la oficina?
7. ¿Tocó Ud. a la víctima?
8. ¿Buscó Ud. a la enfermera?
9. ¿Sacó Ud. el dinero?
10. ¿Atacó Ud. al hombre?

Change the sentences from the present to the preterite tense.

1. Mi marido y yo llegamos tarde.
2. El cirujano me saca las amígdalas.
3. El hombre ataca al policía.
4. El joven se aplica el linimento.
5. Mi padre paga en la oficina.
6. La niña mastica las pastillas.
7. Los médicos me explican el caso.
8. Las enfermeras llegan con el médico.
9. Trago el líquido.
10. Los técnicos buscan a la doctora.

Written practice

Translate the sentences into Spanish.

1. The ambulance arrived quickly.
2. The child swallowed the poison.
3. The woman took an overdose of sleeping pills.
4. They took him away in a stretcher.
5. The neighbors explained what happened to the policeman.
6. He stabbed her with a kitchen knife.
7. The man attacked the woman in the street.
8. They bandaged his leg.
9. I didn't touch the victim.
10. She tried to commit suicide many times.

Grammar

MORE IRREGULAR VERBS IN THE PRETERITE TENSE

decir	dije	dijo	dijo	dijimos	dijeron	dijeron
estar	estuve	estuvo	estuvo	estuvimos	estuvieron	estuvieron
hacer	hice	hizo	hizo	hicimos	hicieron	hicieron
*****poder**	pude	pudo	pudo	pudimos	pudieron	pudieron
poner	puse	puso	puso	pusimos	pusieron	pusieron
*****querer**	quise	quiso	quiso	quisimos	quisieron	quisieron
*****saber**	supe	supo	supo	supimos	supieron	supieron
tener	tuve	tuvo	tuvo	tuvimos	tuvieron	tuvieron
venir	vine	vino	vino	vinimos	vinieron	vinieron

Por fin, la madre pudo hablar con el médico.	*The mother finally managed to speak with the doctor.*
El anciano no quiso ingresar en un hospicio para ancianos.	*The old man refused to enter a nursing home.*
El enfermo supo ayer que tiene cáncer.	*The sick man found out yesterday that he has cancer.*

The verb **conocer** used in the preterite means *to meet.* For example:

Conocí al médico ayer.	*I met the doctor yesterday.*

* Because the preterite specifies a completed past action (and not an ongoing one), some verbs have different meanings when they are used in that tense. In this list the words **poder, querer,** and **saber** are of that type.

Oral practice

Change the sentences using the cues.

1. El médico vino a tiempo.
   • el cura   • la doctora   • las enfermeras   • nosotros
2. El niño dijo la verdad.
   • las muchachas   • la joven   • mi hermano y yo   • la psicóloga
3. No hicimos los ejercicios.
   • yo   • mi abuelo   • el enfermo   • los hombres
4. Mi hermana estuvo enferma anoche.
   • nosotros   • yo   • mi padre   • los niños
5. Las enfermeras les pusieron las inyecciones a las víctimas.
   • los médicos   • la enfermera y yo   • la doctora   • yo

Answer the questions with complete sentences.

1. ¿Qué hizo Ud. para ayudar a la víctima del accidente?
2. ¿Quién le puso la inyección a la víctima?
3. ¿Por qué no quiso el enfermo volver al hospital?
4. ¿Dónde estuvo la madre anoche a las ocho?
5. ¿Por qué no vino Ud. a tiempo?
6. ¿Pudieron Uds. hablar con la víctima del accidente?
7. ¿Supo Ud. por qué atentó el suicidio el joven?
8. ¿Qué le dijo Ud. al policía?
9. ¿Por qué no quiso nadie ayudar al hombre?
10. ¿Supo Ud. la verdad?

Grammar

MORE IRREGULAR VERBS IN THE PRETERITE TENSE

caer	caí	cayó	cayó	caímos	cayeron	cayeron
dar	di	dio	dio	dimos	dieron	dieron
dormir	dormí	durmió	durmió	dormimos	durmieron	durmieron
*****ir**	fui	fue	fue	fuimos	fueron	fueron
leer	leí	leyó	leyó	leímos	leyeron	leyeron
morir	morí	murió	murió	morimos	murieron	murieron
seguir	seguí	siguió	siguió	seguimos	siguieron	siguieron
*****ser**	fui	fue	fue	fuimos	fueron	fueron
ver	vi	vio	vio	vimos	vieron	vieron

* The verbs **ir** and **ser** have the same forms for the preterite.

Oral practice

Change the sentences using the cues.

Fuimos a la sala de emergencia.	*We went to the emergency room.*
La madre del niño fue a la sala de emergencia.	*The child's mother went to the emergency room.*

1. El hombre murió anoche.
   - mi madre   • las víctimas del accidente   • el joven   • la enferma
2. Seguí las instrucciones de la enfermera de ambulancia.
   - nosotros   • el asistente   • el camillero   • los vecinos
3. El muchacho se cayó.
   - las jóvenes   • la anciana   • mi hijo   • yo

Change the sentences from the plural to the singular.

1. Las enfermeras les dieron la medicina a los pacientes.
2. Los niños se cayeron.
3. Los pacientes leyeron los periódicos.
4. Los médicos fueron a la clínica.
5. Seguimos las instrucciones de las enfermeras.
6. Los muchachos vieron lo que pasó.
7. Fuimos a la farmacia anoche.
8. Los pacientes siguieron al técnico al laboratorio.
9. Vimos al paciente en la sala de cuidado intensivo.
10. Mis hermanos murieron en un accidente.

Conversations

A: ¿Qué le pasó a Ud.?
B: Creo que me rompí el brazo.
A: ¿Cómo lo hizo Ud.?
B: Me caí en la cocina y no puedo moverlo.
A: Tendremos que hacer una radiografía del brazo.

A: What happened to you?
B: I think I broke my arm.
A: How did you do it?
B: I fell in the kitchen and I can't move it.
A: We'll have to take an X-ray of the arm.

A: ¿Cómo está su hijo? Me dijeron que sufrió una concusión.
B: Está mejor, gracias, pero nos dio un susto terrible.
A: ¿Cómo ocurrió el accidente?
B: Se cayó en el parque.

A: How is your son? I was told that he suffered a concussion.
B: He is better, thanks, but he gave us a terrible fright.
A: How did the accident happen?
B: He fell in the park.

A: ¿Qué dicen los médicos?

B: Dicen que está fuera de peligro pero tiene que mantenerse quieto y descansar mucho.

A: What do the doctors say?

B: They say that he is out of danger but he must stay still and rest a lot.

Written practice

Translate the sentences into Spanish.

1. Did they have to carry him on a stretcher?
2. What did the policeman say?
3. Did the man die?
4. I explained what happened to the police.
5. They couldn't arrive on time.
6. He swallowed the poison.
7. They gave him artificial respiration.
8. The ambulance brought him in yesterday.
9. The child swallowed poison.
10. The patient suffered a broken leg.

Dialogue

ENFERMERA DE AMBULANCIA: ¿Llamó Ud. por una ambulancia?

VECINO: Sí.

ENFERMERA DE AMBULANCIA: ¿Qué pasó?

VECINO: Mi vecino, el señor Moreno, se cayó escalera abajo y fracturó la pierna. No puede caminar.

ENFERMERA DE AMBULANCIA: ¿Dónde está?

VECINO: Está arriba, en el segundo piso.

SEÑOR MORENO: ¿Ha llegado la ambulancia?

ENFERMERA DE AMBULANCIA: Sí, estamos aquí. ¿Cómo se siente Ud.?

SEÑOR MORENO: Estoy un poco mareado y me duele mucho la pierna.

ENFERMERA DE AMBULANCIA: Vamos a llevarlo a Ud. al hospital en camilla.

(en el hospital)

ENFERMERA: ¿Cómo se llama Ud.?

SEÑOR MORENO: Me llamo Miguel Moreno.

ENFERMERA: ¿Qué le pasó?

SEÑOR MORENO: Me caí escalera abajo en mi casa.

ENFERMERA: ¿Cuándo ocurrió el accidente?

SEÑOR MORENO: Ocurrió hace un par de horas.

ENFERMERA: Vamos a hacer unas radiografías de la pierna.

SEÑOR MORENO: ¿Me va a doler?

ENFERMERA:	No le va a doler. Ud. ha fracturado la pierna y tenemos que llamar al especialista ahora mismo. Él va a enyesar la pierna, y luego se sentirá mejor.
SEÑOR MORENO:	¿Podré caminar?
ENFERMERA:	Ud. tendrá que andar con muletas por unos meses, pero por ahora, tiene que usar una silla de ruedas.

VOCABULARY

la enfermera de ambulancia
  ambulance nurse
el vecino, la vecina *neighbor*
escalera abajo (arriba) *downstairs (upstairs)*
segundo,-a *second*

el piso *floor*
mareado,-a *dizzy*
ahora mismo *right now*
las muletas *crutches*
la silla de ruedas *wheelchair*

AMBULANCE NURSE:	Did you call for an ambulance?
NEIGHBOR:	Yes.
AMBULANCE NURSE:	What happened?
NEIGHBOR:	My neighbor, Mr. Moreno, fell down the stairs and broke his leg. He can't walk.
AMBULANCE NURSE:	Where is he?
NEIGHBOR:	He's upstairs, on the second floor.
MR. MORENO:	Has the ambulance arrived?
AMBULANCE NURSE:	Yes, we're here. How are you feeling?
MR. MORENO:	I'm a bit dizzy and my leg hurts a lot.
AMBULANCE NURSE:	We're going to bring you to the hospital on a stretcher.

(in the hospital)

NURSE:	What is your name?
MR. MORENO:	My name is Miguel Moreno.
NURSE:	What happened to you?
MR. MORENO:	I fell down the stairs in my house.
NURSE:	When did the accident occur?
MR. MORENO:	It occurred a couple of hours ago.
NURSE:	We're going to take some X-rays of your leg.
MR. MORENO:	Is it going to hurt?
NURSE:	It's not going to hurt. You have broken your leg and we have to call the specialist right now. He is going to put the leg in a cast, and later you will feel better.
MR. MORENO:	Will I be able to walk?
NURSE:	You will have to walk with crutches for a few months, but for now, you have to use a wheelchair.

QUESTIONS ON DIALOGUE

1. ¿Qué le pasó al señor Moreno?
2. ¿Quién llamó por la ambulancia?
3. ¿Cómo llevaron al señor Moreno al hospital?
4. ¿Cuándo ocurrió el accidente?
5. ¿Qué hizo la enfermera en el hospital?
6. ¿Quién va a enyesarle la pierna al señor Moreno?
7. ¿Podrá caminar? ¿Cómo?

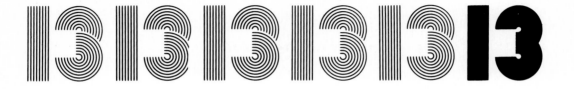

Grammar

IMPERFECT TENSE OF REGULAR VERBS

FIRST CONJUGATION: **hablar**   *to speak;* **yo hablaba**   *I was speaking, I used to speak*

yo	**hablaba**	*I was speaking*
él/ella	**hablaba**	*he/she was speaking*
Ud.	**hablaba**	*you were speaking*
nosotros/nosotras	**hablábamos**	*we were speaking*
ellos/ellas	**hablaban**	*they were speaking*
Uds.	**hablaban**	*you* (pl.) *were speaking*

SECOND CONJUGATION: **comer**   *to eat;* **yo comía**   *I was eating, I used to eat*

yo	**comía**	*I was eating*
él/ella	**comía**	*he/she was eating*
Ud.	**comía**	*you were eating*
nosotros/nosotras	**comíamos**	*we were eating*
ellos/ellas	**comían**	*they were eating*
Uds.	**comían**	*you* (pl.) *were eating*

THIRD CONJUGATION: **escribir**   *to write;* **yo escribía**   *I was writing, I used to write*

yo	**escribía**	*I was writing*
él/ella	**escribía**	*he/she was writing*
Ud.	**escribía**	*you were writing*
nosotros/nosotras	**escribíamos**	*we were writing*
ellos/ellas	**escribían**	*they were writing*
Uds.	**escribían**	*you* (pl.) *were writing*

There are only three verbs that are irregular in the imperfect tense.

ir	iba	iba	iba	íbamos	iban	iban
ser	era	era	era	éramos	eran	eran
ver	veía	veía	veía	veíamos	veían	veían

The imperfect tense is used to indicate something habitual or customary, a repeated action that took place in the past. The most common English equivalents are *used to, would,* and the past progressive (*I was speaking, you were eating,* etc.). For example:

Íbamos a su casa todos los días.	*We would go to his house every day.*
Yo visitaba al enfermo cada día.	*I used to visit the sick man every day.*
El médico hablaba con la enfermera.	*The doctor was speaking with the nurse.*

The imperfect tense is also used to describe feelings, desires, emotions, and state of mind in the past.

La paciente quería ir a casa.	*The patient wanted to go home.*
Ella no sabía que su hijo estaba enfermo.	*She didn't know that her son was ill.*
La paciente tenía miedo.	*The patient was afraid.*
Yo creía que él decía la verdad.	*I believed that he was telling the truth.*
Pensábamos que ella iba a venir.	*We thought that she was going to come.*

It is also used to describe a person, place, situation, or thing in the past.

La joven era linda.	*The young girl was pretty.*
La enfermera era muy simpática.	*The nurse was very nice.*
El hospital era muy grande.	*The hospital was very large.*
La situación era difícil.	*The situation was difficult.*

It is used to indicate time in the past. For example:

| **Eran las dos cuando él me llamó.** | *It was two when he called me.* |

The imperfect forms of **estar** are used with the gerund to form the past progressive tense. For example:

| **¿Qué estaba haciendo Ud.?** | *What were you doing?* |
| **Estaba hablando con el médico.** | *I was speaking with the doctor.* |

It is used with the verb form **hacía** plus a specific time interval to express *had been* plus a gerund. For example:

| **Hacía un mes que vivíamos allí.** | *We had been living there a month.* |

Oral practice

Change the sentences using the cues.

1. La muchacha necesitaba mucho dinero cada semana.
   ● los jóvenes   ● mi hermano   ● mi esposo y yo   ● yo

2. La mujer tomaba la medicina cada día.
   ● los pacientes   ● la muchacha   ● el enfermo   ● mi padre

3. Yo visitaba a mi madre con frecuencia.
   ● mis hermanos   ● mis parientes   ● mi hermana   ● nuestros vecinos

4. La mujer siempre quería visitar al enfermo.
   ● yo   ● mi abuelo   ● la joven   ● mis padres y yo

5. El muchacho hacía los ejercicios todos los días.
   ● los muchachos   ● la paciente   ● mi primo   ● mis amigos y yo

6. Comíamos en la cafetería frecuentemente.
   ● las enfermeras   ● el médico   ● los técnicos   ● la doctora

7. Salíamos temprano del hospital los viernes.
   ● las doctoras   ● el médico   ● yo   ● su esposa

8. Los jóvenes discutían sus problemas cada sábado.
   ● las enfermeras   ● el médico y yo   ● los ancianos   ● las terapistas

9. Yo escribía las cartas cada semana.
   ● la enfermera   ● las muchachas   ● mis hermanas y yo   ● mis padres

Change the sentences from the present to the imperfect tense following the model.

El hombre visita a su hijo ahora.   *The man is visiting his son now.*
El hombre visitaba a su hijo todos   *The man would visit his son every day.*
los días.

1. El paciente come el pan ahora.
2. El farmacéutico prepara la receta ahora.
3. Trabajamos en la clínica ahora.
4. La asistenta hace las camas ahora.
5. Los técnicos hacen los análisis ahora.
6. La mujer visita a su hijo ahora.
7. Los pacientes quieren dormir ahora.
8. Abrimos las ventanas ahora.
9. Las mujeres se bañan ahora.
10. Ellos caminan al hospital ahora.

Change the sentences to the singular.

1. Los hombres iban al hospital cada mes.
2. Las enfermeras iban a la cafetería cada día.
3. Íbamos al hospicio para ancianos cada semana.
4. Los muchachos iban a la casa de su amigo enfermo cada semana.
5. Los técnicos iban al laboratorio cada día.
6. Las mujeres iban al consultorio del médico cada mes.
7. Los farmacéuticos iban a la farmacia cada día.

8. Íbamos a Puerto Rico cada año.
9. Los niños iban a la clínica dental cada seis meses.
10. Íbamos al banco cada semana.

Change the sentences to the plural.

1. El técnico era competente.
2. La enfermera era simpática.
3. La niña era flaca.
4. La madre era irresponsable.
5. El médico era sensible.
6. El hombre era inflexible.
7. El muchacho era alto.
8. La asistenta era antipática.
9. La joven era linda.
10. El niño era inteligente.

Change the sentences from the present to the imperfect tense following the model.

Vemos al médico cada día.   *We see the doctor every day.*
Veíamos al médico cada día.   *We used to see the doctor every day.*

1. Los jóvenes ven al médico cada día.
2. La muchacha ve a la enfermera a menudo.
3. Mi hermano ve a mis padres con frecuencia.
4. Sus padres ven al hombre frecuentemente.
5. La doctora ve al técnico cada semana.
6. Vemos al policía con frecuencia.
7. Yo veo a las terapistas cada semana.
8. La joven ve al bombero a menudo.
9. Veo al farmacéutico cada semana.
10. Mis padres y yo vemos a la muchacha frecuentemente.

Vocabulary

ALCOHOLISM AND DRUG ADDICTION/EL ALCOHOLISMO Y LA NARCOMANIA

el adicto *drug addict*
la aguja hipodérmica *hypodermic needle*
el alcohol *alcohol*
el alcohólico *alcoholic*
el alcoholismo *alcoholism*
la alucinación *hallucination*
alucinador,-a *hallucinatory*
el alucinador *hallucinogen*
alucinante *hallucinating*
alucinar *to hallucinate*
las anfetaminas *amphetamines*
el apetito *appetite*
el aspecto *aspect, appearance, look*

aspirar *to breathe in*
atontado,-a *bewildered, stupified*
aturdido,-a *giddy*
los barbituratos *barbiturates*
los barbitúricos *barbiturates*
la bebida alcohólica *alcoholic beverage*
el calambre *cramp*
el cambio *change*
la cocaína *cocaine*
la codeína *codeine*
el coma *coma*
el comportamiento *behavior*
las consecuencias *consequences*

el consejo profesional *professional counselling*
el criminal *criminal*
el choque nervioso *nervous shock*
decir tonterías *to say foolish things*
deprimido,-a *depressed*
la desintoxicación *detoxification*
desintoxicar *detoxify*
la desnutrición *malnutrition*
desorientado, a *disoriented*
la dosis excesiva *overdose*
las drogas *drugs*
estornudar *to sneeze*
la heroína *heroin*
la inyección hipodérmica *hypodermic injection*
maltratar *to abuse, to maltreat*
el maltrato de los niños *child abuse*
la marihuana *marijuana*

mentir *to lie*
la metadona *methadone*
el narcómano *drug addict*
los narcóticos *narcotics*
los ojos sin brillo *glassy eyes*
perder peso *to lose weight*
los problemas maritales *marital problems*
quedarse en cama *to stay in bed*
respirar con dificultad *to have trouble breathing*
los síntomas *symptoms*
suspender el uso *to stop using (temporarily)*
la suspensión del uso *withdrawal*
tambalear *to stagger*
el tecato *drug addict (slang)*
el tratamiento *treatment*
volar *to fly*

Oral practice

Change the sentences from the imperfect to the preterite tense.

1. La joven tomaba los barbitúricos.
2. Sus amigos fumaban la marihuana.
3. Yo buscaba empleo en la ciudad.
4. El hombre vendía las drogas.
5. Íbamos a la clínica.
6. Mi hermana veía a los otros adictos.
7. El muchacho perdía mucho peso.
8. Salíamos con nuestros amigos.
9. La mujer dormía en la calle.
10. Los jóvenes recibían los tratamientos de metadona.
11. Mi hijo se quedaba en la cama.
12. Nuestro hermano moría de una dosis excesiva de narcóticos.
13. La madre maltrataba a sus hijos.
14. El muchacho decía tonterías.
15. El adicto usaba una aguja hipodérmica.

Written practice

Translate the sentences into Spanish.

1. The young man is sneezing a lot.
2. The addict has respiratory problems.

3. The woman is suffering from malnutrition.
4. The patient has cramps.
5. The young girl is suffering from nervous shock.
6. He was hallucinating and wanted to fly.
7. The boy is vomiting a lot.
8. The addict is suffering from hepatitis.
9. She has glassy eyes.
10. The alcoholic was staggering.
11. The young people were hallucinating.
12. The doctors must detoxify him.
13. The boy was giddy.
14. The addict was having liver and kidney problems.
15. I was quite bewildered.

Grammar

CONTRASTING PRETERITE AND IMPERFECT TENSES

The preterite tense is used to tell what happened; the imperfect tense tells what was happening. For example:

El joven tomó drogas ayer.   *The young man took drugs yesterday.*
El joven tomaba drogas con   *The young man was taking drugs*
  frecuencia.   *frequently.*

The preterite and imperfect tenses are often used in the same sentence. The imperfect might be used to describe what was happening, to describe a scene in the past, while the preterite is used to tell what happened to interrupt that scene. For example:

El paciente dormía cuando la   *The patient was sleeping when the nurse*
  enfermera entró en el cuarto.   *entered the room.*

Oral practice

Change the sentences from the preterite to the imperfect tense following the model.

El muchacho tomó drogas ayer.   *The boy took drugs yesterday.*
El muchacho tomaba drogas a   *The boy was taking drugs often.*
  menudo.

1. El joven usó barbituratos ayer.
2. Mi hermano y yo fuimos a la clínica ayer.
3. Las muchachas visitaron al adicto ayer.
4. Los médicos desintoxicaron al hombre ayer.
5. Mi hermano tomó LSD ayer.
6. El adicto comió poco ayer.
7. Fuimos a la cafetería ayer.

8. La enfermera ayudó al alcohólico ayer.
9. El joven atentó el suicidio ayer.
10. Busqué empleo ayer.

Complete each sentence with the imperfect tense using the cues.

1. Cuando el médico entró en el cuarto el paciente . . .
   • was sleeping   • was doing the exercises   • was watching television   • was taking the medicine   • was talking on the telephone

2. Cuando la doctora entró en el cuarto la enfermera . . .
   • was taking the patient's pulse   • was giving the medicine to the patient   • was washing the patient   • was helping the patient walk   • was giving the patient an injection

3. Cuando yo entré en la farmacia el farmacéutico . . .
   • was selling the medicine   • was preparing the prescription   • was giving some advice to the mother of a sick child   • was explaining something to a customer (*cliente*)   • was talking to the cashier

Conversations

A: ¿Por qué tomó Ud. las anfetaminas?
B: Estaba muy deprimida.
A: ¿Quién se las dio a Ud.?
B: Un amigo de la escuela me las dio.
A: ¿Tomó Ud. algunas anoche?
B: No le voy a decir nada.

A: Why did you take the amphetamines?
B: I was very depressed.
A: Who gave them to you?
B: A friend from school gave them to me.
A: Did you take any last night?
B: I'm not going to tell you anything.

A: Me dijeron que su vecina murió ayer.

B: Sí, tomó barbitúricos y bebidas alcohólicas.
A: ¡Qué lástima! ¿Estaba sola en casa?

B: Lo peor es que su hija de diez años la halló muerta al volver de la escuela.

A: They told me that your neighbor died yesterday.
B: Yes, she took barbiturates and alcohol.
A: What a shame! Was she alone in the house?
B: The worst part is that her ten-year-old daughter found her dead when she returned from school.

A: ¿Por qué se echó de la ventana el joven?
B: Estaba alucinando. Creía que podía volar.
A: ¿Qué drogas estaba tomando?
B: Esta vez tomó LSD.

A: Why did the young man jump out the window?
B: He was hallucinating. He thought that he could fly.
A: What drugs was he taking?
B: This time he took LSD.

A: ¿Qué le pasaba al paciente en el cuarto 450?

A: What was happening to the patient in room 450?

B: Estaba sufriendo de los síntomas de la suspensión del uso de la heroína.

B: He was suffering from withdrawal symptoms from heroin.

A: ¿Dónde tenía dolor?

A: Where was he in pain?

B: Sentía dolor en los músculos y en las articulaciones de las extremidades inferiores. Además, le dolía mucho la cabeza.

B: He was feeling pain in the muscles and the joints of his lower limbs. In addition, he had a bad headache.

A: ¿Por qué tomaba drogas el joven?

A: Why was the young boy taking drugs?

B: Tenía problemas en la escuela y quería escaparse.

B: He was having problems at school and he wanted to escape.

A: ¿Qué hacía cuando Ud. lo visitó?

A: What was he doing when you visited him?

B: Estaba diciendo tonterías. Estaba aturdido y tenía los ojos sin brillo.

B: He was saying silly things. He was giddy and his eyes were glassy.

A: ¿Notó Ud. algún otro cambio en su aspecto?

A: Did you notice any other change in his appearance?

B: Sí, ha perdido peso últimamente.

B: Yes, he has lost weight recently.

A: ¿Por qué tomaba tanto el hombre?

A: Why was the man drinking so much?

B: Tenía problemas maritales.

B: He was having marital problems.

A: ¿Buscaba consejo profesional?

A: Did he seek professional counselling?

B: No, me dijo que no necesitaba la ayuda de nadie.

B: No, he told me that he didn't need anyone's help.

A: ¿Es alcohólico?

A: Is he an alcoholic?

B: No sé por cierto, pero sospecho que sí.

B: I don't know for certain, but I suspect that he is.

Written practice

Translate the sentences into English.

1. Usaba los barbitúricos porque no podía dormir y estaba muy nerviosa.
2. Tomó una dosis excesiva anoche y ahora está en un estado de coma.
3. El adicto era agresivo y anoche atacó a su hermano.
4. Lo llevaron al hospital en una ambulancia.
5. A los jóvenes les gusta usar la cocaína.

Translate the sentences into Spanish.

1. The addict is suffering from withdrawal symptoms from the drug.
2. He needed a lot of money to buy the drugs.
3. He lied about where he was going.

4. Her parents were very worried about her state of health.
5. What did his parents do when they found out that he was an addict?
6. She was very depressed for a long time.
7. She refused to seek professional counselling.
8. Her father was an alcoholic and he abused her mother.
9. Did you notice any changes in your daughter's behavior?
10. Why didn't you help him when he needed you?

Dialogue

SEÑORA: Perdone, doctora, ¿puedo hablar con Ud.?
DOCTORA: Sí, por supuesto. ¿Cuál es su problema, señora?
SEÑORA: Creo que mi hijo toma drogas.
DOCTORA: ¿Por qué cree Ud. eso?
SEÑORA: Pues, anoche, volvió muy tarde a casa, decía tonterías, y no sabía dónde estaba.
DOCTORA: Posiblemente estaba borracho.
SEÑORA: No, a veces mi marido viene a casa borracho y no es lo mismo.
DOCTORA: ¿Tiene Ud. alguna idea de qué drogas tomó anoche?
SEÑORA: Yo sé que mi hijo fumaba marihuana hacía algunos meses, pero creo que lo de anoche fue diferente. Creo que alucinaba.
DOCTORA: Quizás tomó LSD. Ud. debe averiguar si tomaba otras drogas también. Y si toma drogas más fuertes ahora, como la mescalina, el opio, o la heroína, puede ser muy peligroso para su hijo. ¿Halló Ud. alguna vez píldoras en su casa o en el cuarto de su hijo?
SEÑORA: No. ¿Por qué?
DOCTORA: Porque las píldoras como los barbitúricos, las anfetaminas y otras son muy malas. Ud. debe llevar a su hijo aquí para un examen físico.
SEÑORA: Sí. Creo que Ud. tiene razón, doctora. Muchas gracias por su ayuda.

VOCABULARY

perdone *pardon*
por supuesto *of course*
anoche *last night*
posiblemente *possibly*
borracho,-a *drunk*
a veces *sometimes*
lo mismo *the same*

quizás *perhaps*
averiguar *to find out*
el opio *opium*
la mescalina *mescaline*
peligroso,-a *dangerous*
hallar *to find*
tener razón *to be right*

WOMAN: Pardon, doctor, can I speak with you?
DOCTOR: Yes, of course. What is your problem, ma'am?
WOMAN: I think that my son is taking drugs.
DOCTOR: Why do you think that?

WOMAN: Well, last night, he returned home very late, was saying crazy things, and didn't know where he was.

DOCTOR: It's possible that he was drunk.

WOMAN: No, sometimes my husband comes home drunk and it's not the same.

DOCTOR: Do you have any idea what drugs he took?

WOMAN: I know that my son had been smoking marijuana a few months ago, but I believe that last night's incident was different. I believe that he was hallucinating.

DOCTOR: Perhaps he took LSD. You should find out if he was taking other drugs also. And if he's taking stronger drugs now, like mescaline, opium, or heroin, it can be very dangerous for your son. Did you ever find pills in your house or in your son's room?

WOMAN: No. Why?

DOCTOR: Because pills like barbiturates, amphetamines, and others are very bad. You should bring your son in for a physical examination.

WOMAN: Yes. I believe that you are right, doctor. Thank you very much for your help.

QUESTIONS ON DIALOGUE

1. ¿Cuál es el problema de la señora?
2. ¿Por qué cree ella que su hijo toma drogas?
3. ¿Cómo sabe ella que su hijo no estaba borracho?
4. ¿Qué droga tomaba su hijo hacía algunos meses?
5. ¿Por qué fue diferente lo de anoche?
6. ¿Cuáles son algunos ejemplos de drogas fuertes?
7. Según la doctora, ¿qué debe hacer la señora?

ANALYSIS OF DIALOGUE

1. ¿Cree Ud. que la señora tiene razón al solicitar la ayuda de la doctora?
2. Según la información que le da la señora a la doctora, ¿cree Ud. que su hijo toma drogas?
3. ¿Cree Ud. que un examen físico es una buena idea? ¿Qué indicará un examen físico?

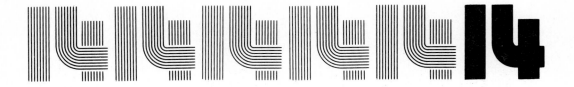

Grammar

COMPARISON OF ADJECTIVES

eficaz	*effective*	**el más (menos) eficaz**	
más eficaz	*more effective*	**la más (menos) eficaz**	the most
menos eficaz	*less effective*	**los más (menos) eficaces**	(least)
		las más (menos) eficaces	effective

For comparison of adjectives we simply use the words **más,** meaning *more,* and **menos,** meaning *less.* For the superlative we use the definite article with **más** or **menos.** The definite article (along with the adjective) must agree in gender and number with the noun. Some comparisons are irregular. For example:

bueno	*good*	**malo**	*bad*
mejor	*better*	**peor**	*worse*
el mejor	*best*	**el peor**	*worst*

In comparisons, the word *than* is translated by **que.**

> **La heroína es peor que la marihuana.** *Heroin is worse than marijuana.*

Comparisons of equality use the words **tan . . . como,** which are the equivalent of the English *as . . . as.* For example:

> **La medicina es tan eficaz como el ungüento.** *The medicine is as effective as the ointment.*

Vocabulary

CONTRACEPTION/LA CONTRACEPCIÓN

el anillo *ring*
los aparatos intrauterinos *intrauterine devices*

el condón *condom*
las cremas vaginales *vaginal creams*
el diafragma *diaphragm*

la ducha *douche*
el escudo *shield*
el esperma *sperm*
el espiral *spiral*
las espumas *foams*
la esterilización *sterilization*
el gorro cervical *cervical cap*
el huevo *egg*
la jalea *jelly*
los lavados vaginales *douches*
el lazo *loop*

la ligadura de los tubos *tubal ligation*
el método anticonceptivo *method of contraception*
el método de ritmo *rhythm method*
el nudo *bow*
la píldora *the pill*
el profiláctico *prophylactic*
las relaciones sexuales *sexual relations*
la retirada *withdrawal*
la vasectomía *vasectomy*

Oral practice

Answer the questions by following the model.

¿Es el profiláctico tan eficaz como la espuma?

Is the prophylactic as effective as the foam?

No, el profiláctico es más eficaz que la espuma.

No, the prophylactic is more effective than the foam.

1. ¿Es la píldora tan eficaz como el ritmo?
2. ¿Es el lazo tan eficaz como la ducha?
3. ¿Es el condón tan eficaz como la retirada?
4. ¿Es el diafragma tan eficaz como el lavado vaginal?
5. ¿Es el nudo tan eficaz como la jalea?

Answer the questions with complete sentences.

1. Entre la jalea, la crema vaginal, y la espuma, ¿cuál es el mejor método anticonceptivo? ¿cuál es el peor?
2. Entre el lazo, el espiral, y el nudo, ¿cuál es el aparato intrauterino más eficaz? ¿cuál es el menos eficaz?
3. Entre el ritmo, el anillo, y el diafragma, ¿cuál es el método anticonceptivo más seguro? ¿cuál es el menos seguro? ¿Es el ritmo mejor que el anillo? ¿Es el diafragma peor que el anillo?
4. Entre el profiláctico, el gorro cervical, y la píldora, ¿cuál es el método anticonceptivo más peligroso? ¿Es el primero más peligroso que el segundo?
5. ¿Es el escudo tan eficaz como el diafragma? ¿Cuál es el método anticonceptivo más seguro?

Conversations

METHODS OF CONTRACEPTION

A: Estoy interesada en usar la píldora como método anticonceptivo. ¿Puede Ud. darme alguna información sobre ella?

A: I'm interested in using the pill as a method of contraception. Can you give me some information on it?

B: ¿Qué quiere saber?

A: ¿Es muy eficaz?

B: Sí, es un método anticonceptivo muy eficaz.

A: ¿Cuándo debo tomar las píldoras?

B: Ud. tiene que tomar una píldora cada día.

A: ¿Necesito una receta para comprarlas?

B: Claro que sí.

B: What do you want to know?

A: Is it very effective?

B: Yes, it is a very effective method of contraception.

A: When must I take the pills?

B: You have to take one pill every day.

A: Do I need a prescription to buy them?

B: Yes, of course.

A: Doctor, hace unos meses que tomo la píldora como método anticonceptivo y he experimentado algunas complicaciones.

B: ¿Cuáles son las complicaciones que Ud. ha experimentado?

A: Tengo las piernas hinchadas y estoy perdiendo el pelo.

B: Ud. debe dejar de usar la píldora.

A: Doctor, I have been taking the pill for a few months as a method of contraception and I've experienced some complications.

B: What are some of the complications that you have experienced?

A: My legs are swollen and I'm losing my hair.

B: You should stop using the pill.

A: Doctor, estoy interesada en usar el diafragma para el control de la natalidad. ¿Es un método bueno?

B: Sí. Es fácil de usar y es relativamente eficaz.

A: ¿Qué debo hacer para usar este método?

B: Yo debo determinar el tamaño correcto para Ud., ya que no todas las mujeres usan el mismo tamaño de diafragma.

A: ¿Es todo, doctor?

B: Le voy a mostrar cómo insertar el diafragma, porque Ud. tiene que hacer esto por sí misma antes de tener relaciones sexuales.

A: Doctor, I'm interested in using the diaphragm for birth control. Is it a good method?

B: Yes. It's easy to use and it's relatively effective.

A: What do I have to do to use this method?

B: I must determine the correct size for you since not all women use the same size diaphragm.

A: Is that all, doctor?

B: I'm going to show you how to insert the diaphragm, because you have to do this yourself before having sexual relations.

A: Quiero usar el método de ritmo para el control de la natalidad. ¿Es un método eficaz?

B: Es bastante eficaz cuando uno lo comprende correctamente.

A: ¿Qué debo saber para usar este método correctamente?

A: I wish to use the rhythm method as a method of birth control. Is it an effective method?

B: It is fairly effective when properly understood.

A: What should I know in order to use this method correctly?

B: Debemos determinar cuándo es su período fértil y Ud. debe abstenerse de las relaciones sexuales durante este período y unos días antes y después.

A: ¿Puede salir mal este método?

B: Sí. Si su período es irregular durante un mes, entonces Ud. puede embarazarse. Por eso, Ud. debe usar un condón para protección adicional.

B: We must determine when you are fertile and you should abstain from sexual relations during this period and a few days before and after.

A: Can anything go wrong with this method?

B: Yes. If your period is irregular one month, you can become pregnant. For this reason, you should use a condom for additional protection.

Vocabulary

PREGNANCY/EL EMBARAZO

el aborto accidental   *miscarriage*
el aborto provocado   *abortion*
el aborto terapéutico   *therapeutic abortion*
las almorranas   *piles*
alrededor de   *around*
la anemia   *anemia*
la anestesia caudal   *caudal anesthesia*
la anestesia general   *general anesthesia*
la anestesia local   *local anesthetic*
anestesiar   *to anesthetize*
el anestesiólogo   *anesthesiologist*
la bolsa de aguas   *bag of waters*
los calambres   *cramps*
la comadrona   *midwife*
las complicaciones   *complications*
las contracciones   *contractions*
el cordón umbilical   *umbilical cord*
la criatura   *infant*
el cuello uterino   *cervix*
dar a luz   *to give birth*
dar el pecho   *to breastfeed*
los defectos de nacimiento   *birth defects*
la dilatación del cuello uterino   *dilation of the cervix*
los dolores del parto   *labor pains*
los efectos secundarios   *side effects*

los ejercicios de respiración   *breathing exercises*
el embarazo   *pregnancy*
empujar   *to push*
un espinal   *a spinal*
estar de parto   *to be in labor*
estar embarazada   *to be pregnant*
estar encinta   *to be pregnant*
estar en estado   *to be pregnant*
estar preñada   *to be pregnant*
el feto   *fetus*
el flujo de sangre   *discharge of blood*
el fórceps   *forceps*
los gemelos   *twins*
el ginecólogo, la ginecóloga   *gynecologist*
la hemorragia   *hemorrhage*
la incubadora   *incubator*
la inyección intravenosa   *intravenous injection*
el mareo   *dizziness*
la maternidad   *maternity, motherhood*
la menstruación   *menstruation*
nacer   *to be born*
el nacimiento   *birth*
la náusea   *nausea*
las náuseas del embarazo   *morning sickness*
el nene, la nena   *infant*

la obstetricia   *obstetrics*
el obstétrico, la obstétrica
   obstetrician
la operación cesárea   *caesarean*
   operation
la partera   *midwife*
el parto   *childbirth*
el parto múltiple   *multiple childbirth*
el parto natural   *natural childbirth*
el parto prematuro   *premature birth*
el pentotal sódico   *sodium pentothal*
el período   *menstrual period*

pesar   *to weigh*
la presión alta   *high blood pressure*
la prueba del embarazo   *pregnancy*
   test
la regla   *menstrual period*
la sala de partos   *delivery room*
la toxemia   *toxemia*
violar   *to rape*
los vómitos del embarazo   *morning*
   sickness

Conversations

PAST PREGNANCIES

A: ¿Es su primer embarazo?
B: No, es mi segundo.
A: ¿Ha tenido Ud. abortos?
B: No, no he tenido ningún aborto.
A: ¿Tuvo Ud. problemas con el primer embarazo?
B: Sí, tuvieron que efectuar una operación cesárea.

A: Is this your first pregnancy?
B: No, it's my second.
A: Have you had any abortions?
B: No, I haven't had any.
A: Did you have any problems with your first pregnancy?
B: Yes, they had to perform a caesarean operation.

A: ¿Ha tenido Ud. partos múltiples?
B: Sí, di a luz a gemelos.
A: ¿Ha usado Ud. contraceptivos?
B: Sí, he usado la píldora pero ya no.

A: Have you had multiple births?
B: Yes, I gave birth to twins.
A: Have you used contraceptives?
B: Yes, I've used the pill, but I'm no longer using it.

A: ¿Cuándo dejó Ud. de usar la píldora?
B: Hace seis meses.

A: When did you stop using the pill?
B: Six months ago.

A: ¿Tuvo Ud. problemas con el primer embarazo?
B: Sí, mi bebé nació con defectos de nacimiento.
A: ¿Cómo ocurrió eso?
B: Tuve rubéola durante el embarazo. embarazo.

A: Did you have problems with your first pregnancy?
B: Yes, my baby was born with birth defects.
A: How did that happen?
B: I had rubella during the pregnancy.

A: ¿Tuvo Ud. problemas con el primer embarazo?

A: Did you have any problems with the first pregnancy?

B: Sí, fue un parto prematuro. Mi nena tuvo que quedarse en una incubadora.

A: ¿Cuánto pesó ella al nacer?

B: Cinco libras.

B: Yes, it was a premature birth. My baby had to stay in an incubator.

A: How much did she weigh at birth?

B: Five pounds.

Written practice

Translate the sentences into English.

1. El obstétrico tuvo que usar fórceps.
2. ¿Cuál fue el problema con su primer embarazo?
3. Mi nene nació con el cordón umbilical alrededor del cuello.
4. Los gemelos nacieron con defectos de nacimiento.
5. Tuvieron que meter la criatura en una incubadora.
6. La obstétrica recomendó una operación cesárea.
7. A los siete meses la mujer tuvo un aborto accidental.
8. Le dieron la anestesia general a la mujer.
9. Fue un parto natural.
10. El anestesiólogo le dio una inyección intravenosa a la mujer.

Cued situation

MEDICAL HISTORY AND PAST PREGNANCIES

You are the obstetrician and you must ask the expectant mother the following questions with the help of the vocabulary below.

VOCABULARY

el cáncer *cancer*
la diabetis *diabetes*
las enfermedades del corazón *heart disease*
las enfermedades de los riñones *kidney disease*
las enfermedades venéreas *venereal disease*

la escarlatina *scarlet fever*
la fiebre reumática *rheumatic fever*
las paperas *mumps*
la pulmonía *pneumonia*
la rubéola *rubella*
el sarampión *measles*
la tuberculosis *tuberculosis*

1. Has she ever suffered from heart disease, kidney disease, venereal disease, scarlet fever, rheumatic fever, mumps, pneumonia, measles, or tuberculosis?

2. Has any member of her family ever suffered from cancer, diabetes, heart disease, or kidney disease?

3. Has she ever been pregnant before and if so, what significant problems (if any) did she have during the pregnancies?

Conversations

PRESENT PREGNANCY

A: Creo que estoy en estado.

B: ¿Cómo sabe Ud. esto?

A: Bueno, hace dos meses que no tengo la regla. Además, tengo náuseas por la mañana y vómitos también.

B: ¿Ha consultado Ud. con su obstétrico?

A: Todavía no, pero pienso hacerlo pronto.

A: La joven fue violada y ahora está encinta.

B: ¿Va a tener un aborto?

A: Sí, según la ley tiene el derecho a tener un aborto terapéutico.

B: ¿Qué dicen sus padres?

A: Están a favor de la decisión.

A: I think I'm pregnant.

B: How do you know that?

A: Well, I haven't had my period for two months. Besides, I have morning sickness.

B: Have you consulted with your obstetrician?

A: Not yet, but I intend to do so soon.

A: The young girl was raped and now she is pregnant.

B: Is she going to have an abortion?

A: Yes, according to the law she has the right to a therapeutic abortion.

B: What do her parents say?

A: They are in favor of the decision.

Written practice

Translate the sentences into English.

1. Tengo flujo de sangre.
2. Voy a darle el pecho al nene.
3. Me duelen los pechos.
4. La paciente tiene almorranas.
5. Tengo problemas con la visión.
6. ¿Cuándo va a dar a luz?
7. La mujer tiene rubéola y está embarazada.
8. Tiene vómitos por la mañana.
9. Necesita la ayuda de una partera.
10. Tiene que visitar al obstétrico.

Role playing

One student takes the role of the obstetrician and must ask the patient if she has been suffering from the following symptoms during her pregnancy:

1. problems with her vision
2. dizziness
3. nausea
4. vomiting
5. discharge of blood
6. others

The student playing the role of the pregnant woman tells the obstetrician that she is suffering from the above and has the following problems and questions:

1. She has to work because she doesn't have enough money.
2. She comes home very tired from work.
3. She always feels tired.
4. Should she stop working?

Conversations

LABOR AND DELIVERY

A: ¿Cómo se siente Ud.?

B: Tengo mucho dolor. Me duele la espalda y tengo calambres.

A: ¿Quiere tomar algo para aliviar el dolor?

B: No estoy segura. ¿Qué puedo tomar?

A: Podemos darle un sedante, ponerle una inyección o a lo mejor le podemos anestesiar.

A: ¿Se ha preparado Ud. para el parto natural?

B: Sí.

A: Entonces, trate de calmarse con los ejercicios de respiración. Las enfermeras y su marido están aquí para ayudarle.

B: Gracias, doctor. Si tengo mucho dolor, ¿me puede dar algo para aliviarlo?

A: Sí. Si es necesario podemos ponerle una inyección.

A: How are you feeling?

B: I'm in a lot of pain. My back hurts and I have cramps.

A: Would you like to take something to relieve the pain?

B: I'm not sure. What can I take?

A: We can give you a sedative, an injection, or perhaps we can anesthetize you.

A: Have you taken the natural childbirth preparation?

B: Yes.

A: Then try to relax with the breathing exercises. The nurses and your husband are here to help you.

B: Thank you, doctor. If I'm in a lot of pain, can you give me something to relieve it?

A: Yes. If it is necessary, we can give you an injection.

Written practice

Translate the sentences into English.

1. El anestesiólogo le puso la inyección a la mujer.
2. Tuvo que respirar profundamente.
3. Fue un parto inducido.
4. La paciente estaba en la sala de partos.
5. Ella tiene las contracciones cada cinco minutos.
6. La paciente prefiere la anestesia general.

7. Se ha roto la bolsa de aguas.
8. La doctora recomendó una operación cesárea.
9. Me dieron un sedante.
10. Anestesiaron a la mujer.

Cued situation

LABOR AND DELIVERY

You are the obstetrician and the expectant mother is about to give birth. You are going to give her the following information and directives and ask her the following questions:

1. Since you are fully dilated now, we are going to take you from the Labor Room to the Delivery Room.

2. When you feel a contraction, breathe in, hold your breath, and bear down.

3. Are you ready? We'll count 1, 2, 3, 4, 5—push!

4. Relax, now—once again.

5. Look, the little head is beginning to emerge, now a shoulder. It's a girl!

Reading

PREGNANCY

Una mujer puede tomar ciertas medidas para determinar con seguridad si está embarazada. Hoy día puede darse a sí misma una prueba del embarazo en su propia casa. Estas pruebas se pueden conseguir en cualquier farmacia. Sin embargo, una mujer que cree que está embarazada debe visitar al médico. De esta manera puede tener una prueba más segura del embarazo. También puede recibir los consejos del médico sobre el cuidado prenatal si está encinta de veras.

VOCABULARY

tomar ciertas medidas *to take certain steps*
determinar *to determine*
con seguridad *with certainty*
conseguir *to get, obtain*
cualquier *any*
de esta manera *in this way*
seguro,-a *sure, certain*
el consejo *advice*
el cuidado prenatal *prenatal care*

QUESTIONS ON READING

1. ¿Cuáles son algunas medidas que una mujer debe tomar para determinar si está encinta?
2. ¿Dónde se pueden conseguir las pruebas del embarazo que se dan en casa?
3. ¿Por qué debe ir al médico la mujer encinta?
4. ¿Qué puede darle el médico?

Written practice

Translate the sentences into Spanish.

1. She has to visit her obstetrician.
2. She is going to give herself a pregnancy test at home.
3. She is going to the pharmacy to buy a pregnancy test.
4. She needs advice on prenatal care.
5. She wants to determine with certainty that she is pregnant.
6. The doctor is going to give her a complete physical examination.
7. He has received the results of the tests.
8. She knows for certain that she is pregnant and intends to tell her husband tonight.
9. The doctor has to ask her a lot of questions.
10. She has to visit the doctor again in a month to check on her condition.

Reading

PREGNANCY

La mujer encinta debe precaucionarse contra posibles complicaciones durante el embarazo porque es muy fácil hacerle daño al feto. Ella debe evitar el uso de las drogas con excepción de aquéllas recetadas por su médico. Debe dejar de fumar y tomar bebidas alcohólicas durante este tiempo, y también debe evitar la actividad estrenua.

Si una mujer está encinta, debe seguir una dieta balanceada y tomar muchas comidas ricas en la proteína como el queso, la leche, los huevos, y el pescado y debe comer frutas y vegetales frescos. Ella también tiene que visitar a su obstétrico regularmente. Le dará a ella un examen médico en que la pesará, le registrará el pulso, le hará un urinálisis, y verificará el desarrollo del feto. Además, el médico determinará si la mujer está experimentando ciertas dificultades o complicaciones como la toxemia que puede atribuirse al exceso de los fluidos en la sangre.

VOCABULARY

precaucionarse *to take precautions*
durante *during*
hacerle daño (a uno) *to hurt, harm*
evitar *avoid*
con excepción de *with the exception of*
aquéllos,-as *those*
recetado,-a *prescribed*
dejar de *to stop*
la actividad estrenua *strenuous activity*

una dieta balanceada *a balanced diet*
las comidas *meals, foods*
rico,-a *rich*
pesar *to weigh*
verificar *to check on*
el desarrollo *development*
experimentar *to experience*
atribuirse a *to be attributed to*
el exceso *excess*
los fluidos *fluids*

QUESTIONS ON READING

1. ¿Cómo puede la mujer encinta hacerle daño al feto?
2. ¿Cuáles son algunas cosas que puede hacer la mujer encinta para evitar ciertas complicaciones en el embarazo?
3. ¿Qué tipo de dieta debe seguir ella?
4. ¿Por qué tiene que visitar al médico regularmente?
5. ¿Qué determinará el médico?

Written practice

Translate the sentences into Spanish.

1. She is taking drugs that are not prescribed by her doctor.
2. These drugs can harm the fetus.
3. She refused to stop smoking and drinking during the pregnancy.
4. The patient had to follow a balanced diet.
5. These foods are high in protein.
6. She is drinking a lot of milk and eating a lot of fresh fruit and vegetables.
7. She hasn't been visiting the obstetrician regularly.
8. The fetus is developing normally.
9. The doctor is giving her a urinalysis.
10. There is an excess of fluid in the blood.

Reading

CHILDBIRTH

Hay varios métodos de parto. La mujer encinta, bajo el consejo de su obstétrico, debe escoger el mejor método para sí misma. En todo caso, debe solicitar la ayuda de un médico, una enfermera o una partera, preferiblemente en un hospital.

Un método de parto natural se llama Lamaze. La mujer trata de relajarse por medio de un conjunto de ejercicios de respiración. Según este método, no se usan drogas (o se usan pocas). De esta manera ni la madre ni el bebé experimentan las complicaciones que pueden ocurrir cuando se usa la anestesia. Además, la madre no sufrirá ciertos efectos secundarios que a veces resultan del uso de la anestesia. Tanto la madre como el padre pueden participar activamente en un momento significante de su vida—el nacimiento de su bebé.

Conforme al método tradicional de parto, se usan drogas como Demerol (primariamente para los dolores del parto), y varios tipos de anestesia como la anestesia general (para el parto), la anestesia caudal, la anestesia local (al momento del parto), o la espinal (generalmente para una sección cesárea). La madre no participa en los pasos preparativos para el parto. El médico se encarga de toda la responsabilidad. La ventaja más grande es que la madre siente el menor dolor posible.

VOCABULARY

el parto *delivery*
bajo *under*
escoger *to choose*
solicitar *to ask for, seek*
la ayuda *help*
preferiblemente *preferably*
tratar de *to try to*
relajarse *relax*
por medio de *by means of*
un conjunto *a set*
los ejercicios de respiración
  breathing exercises

según *according to*
ni . . . ni *neither . . . nor*
el bebé *baby, infant*
ocurrir *to occur*
los efectos secundarios *side effects*
resultar *to result*
tanto . . . como *as well as*
participar *to participate*
los pasos preparativos *preparations*
la ventaja *advantage*

QUESTIONS ON READING

1. ¿Cómo debe una mujer escoger el método de parto más apropiado?
2. Según el método de parto natural, ¿cómo puede relajarse la mujer encinta?
3. ¿Cuáles son algunas ventajas de no usar drogas para el parto?
4. ¿Cuáles son algunos tipos de anestesia que se pueden dar a la mujer encinta para el parto?
5. ¿Cuál es la ventaja más grande del método tradicional de parto?

Written practice

Translate the sentences into Spanish.

1. She wants to choose the best method.
2. She must ask for the help of a midwife.
3. The breathing exercises are important.
4. Certain respiratory problems can occur.
5. The husband will help his wife during the delivery.
6. She doesn't want to use any drugs.
7. What type of anesthesia does your doctor recommend?
8. I want to feel as little pain as possible.
9. She is suffering from certain side effects of the drugs.
10. They are going to give her a spinal for the caesarian operation.

Dialogue

DOCTORA: Los resultados que acaban de llegar del laboratorio indican que Ud. está encinta.
SEÑORITA: No puedo cuidar a un niño.
DOCTORA: ¿Cuántos años tiene Ud.?
SEÑORITA: Tengo solamente diez y ocho años y no tengo dinero.

DOCTORA: ¿Es Ud. casada?

SEÑORITA: No, soy soltera, y mi novio no tiene trabajo.

DOCTORA: Si la criatura es adoptada, todo se arreglará.

SEÑORITA: No, no quiero seguir con el embarazo. Mis padres me botarán de casa.

DOCTORA: Entonces, ¿Ud. vive con sus padres?

SEÑORITA: Sí, y mis padres no querrán problemas como éste. No son muy tolerantes.

DOCTORA: Pues, si Ud. quiere un aborto, debe tenerlo cuanto antes. Ud. está en el segundo mes del embarazo y después de tres meses, según la ley, no se puede tener un aborto.

SEÑORITA: ¿Me va a costar mucho dinero?

DOCTORA: Si va a un médico privado, le costará como trescientos o cuatrocientos dólares. Pero también hay clínicas que ofrecen este servicio.

SEÑORITA: ¿Puede Ud. recomendar una de estas clínicas?

DOCTORA: Por supuesto. Le daré toda la información necesaria.

VOCABULARY

los resultados *results*
cuidar *to take care of*
soltero,-a *single*
el novio *boyfriend*
la novia *girlfriend*
botar *to throw out*
adoptado,-a *adopted*

arreglar *to fix, arrange, resolve*
tolerante *tolerant*
cuanto antes *right away*
según *according to*
la ley *the law*
por supuesto *of course*

DOCTOR: The results that have just come from the lab indicate that you are pregnant.

WOMAN: I can't take care of a child.

DOCTOR: How old are you?

WOMAN: I'm only eighteen years old and I don't have any money.

DOCTOR: Are you married?

WOMAN: No, I'm single and my boyfriend doesn't have a job.

DOCTOR: If the child is adopted, everything will be solved.

WOMAN: No, I don't want to continue with the pregnancy. My parents will throw me out of the house.

DOCTOR: Well then, you live with your parents?

WOMAN: Yes, and my parents won't want problems like this one. They're not very tolerant.

DOCTOR: Well, if you want an abortion, you should have one as soon as possible. You are in the second month of your pregnancy and after three months, according to the law, you can't have an abortion.

WOMAN: Is it going to cost me a lot of money?

DOCTOR: If you go to a private doctor, it will cost you about three or four hundred dollars. But there are also clinics which offer this service.

WOMAN: Can you recommend one of these clinics?

DOCTOR: Of course. I'll give you all the necessary information.

QUESTIONS ON DIALOGUE

1. ¿Qué indican los resultados que acaban de llegar del laboratorio?
2. ¿Cuántos años tiene la señorita?
3. ¿Tiene trabajo su novio?
4. ¿Cómo son los padres de la señorita?
5. ¿En qué mes del embarazo está ella?
6. ¿Cuánto cuesta un aborto?
7. ¿A dónde va esta señorita para el aborto?

ANALYSIS OF DIALOGUE

1. ¿Qué le ha impulsado a la señorita a tomar la decisión del aborto?
2. En su opinión, ¿existen otras alternativas que el aborto para esta mujer?
3. ¿Qué piensa Ud. de la actitud de los padres en este caso?
4. ¿Debe el novio ser responsable del problema también?

QUESTIONS FOR DISCUSSION

1. ¿Cómo se puede evitar el problema del embarazo no deseado?
2. ¿Está Ud. a favor del aborto o no?

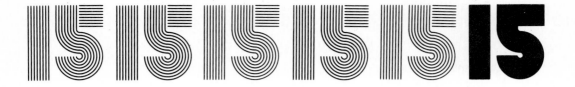

Vocabulary

POSTNATAL CARE/EL CUIDADO POSTNATAL

alimentar   *to feed*
antes de   *before*
el bebé   *baby*
la criatura   *infant*
el biberón   *baby bottle*
cambiar el pañal   *change the diaper*
el cuarto   *room*
dar el pecho   *breastfeed*
dar un baño   *to give a bath*
ensuciar   *to dirty, soil*
esterilizar   *sterilize*
la farmacia   *pharmacy*
la fórmula   *formula*

el lavaplatos   *dishwasher*
lavar   *to wash*
limpiar   *to clean*
el nene   *baby*
la nena   *baby*
el pañal de tela   *cloth diaper*
el pañal desechable   *disposable diaper*
el (la) pediatra   *pediatrician*
la pediatría   *pediatrics*
el pezón de biberón   *nipple of bottle*
preparar   *to prepare*
probar la leche   *to test the milk*
el talco   *talcum powder*

Oral practice

Answer the questions using the vocabulary list on postnatal care.

1. ¿Cuál es la bebida que la madre prepara para el bebé?
2. ¿Qué se tiene que hacer al biberón antes de dárselo al bebé?
3. ¿Cómo se llama la ropa interior que lleva el bebé?
4. Cuando el niño se ensucia, ¿qué tiene que hacer la madre?
5. ¿Qué se le pone al bebé después de darle un baño?
6. ¿Cuál es el médico que se especializa en niños?
7. ¿Qué se tiene que hacer con la fórmula antes de dársela al bebé?
8. ¿Dónde se compran las drogas y otras necesidades para la salud?

Change the sentences by following the models.

Ella le alimenta al bebé ahora.	*She is feeding the baby now.*
Ella le alimentó al bebé ayer.	*She fed the baby yesterday.*
Ella le alimentaba al bebé cada día.	*She used to feed the baby every day.*
Ella le alimentará al bebé mañana.	*She will feed the baby tomorrow.*

1. El padre prepara el cuarto para el bebé.
2. Los padres limpian el cuarto.
3. La madre esteriliza los biberones y los pezones.
4. La hija pone los biberones en el lavaplatos.
5. La madre le da el pecho al bebé.
6. El padre prepara la fórmula.
7. La madre le da un baño a la criatura.
8. La madre usa pañales de tela.
9. El hijo compra pañales desechables.
10. La abuela le cambia el pañal al nene.
11. La madre compra el talco para el bebé.
12. El padre lleva a la nena a la pediatra.
13. La madre prueba la leche antes de dársela al nene.
14. La madre va a la farmacia para comprar la medicina para la criatura.
15. El padre le da la medicina a la nena.

Written practice

Translate the sentences into Spanish.

1. The parents must prepare the formula for the baby.
2. The baby's room is quite warm.
3. The mother should sterilize the nipple and the bottle each time that she uses them.
4. It is beneficial to breastfeed the baby.
5. The parents should bathe the baby often.
6. She prefers to use disposable diapers because she doesn't have the time to wash cloth diapers.
7. After changing the diaper you should put talcum powder on the baby.
8. She tests the milk before she gives it to her baby.
9. I must make an appointment with the pediatrician.
10. I'm going to change the baby's diaper because she has had a bowel movement.

Vocabulary

CHILDHOOD AILMENTS AND ACCIDENTS
DOLENCIAS Y ACCIDENTES DE LA INFANCIA

la anemia *anemia*
el agua hirviente *boiling water*
atragantarse *to choke*

beber *to drink*
caerse de *to fall from*
cólico *colic*

el cuchillo   *knife*
digerir   *to digest*
dormir   *to sleep*
el eczema   *eczema*
echarse gases   *to expel gas*
eliminar   *to defecate*
enfermarse   *to become ill*
eructar   *to belch*
la escaldadura   *diaper rash*
el salpullido   *diaper rash*
estar estreñido,-a   *to be constipated*
flaco   *slender, skinny*
hacerse daño   *to harm oneself*
el impétigo   *impetigo*
llorar   *to cry*

molestar   *to bother*
padecer de   *to suffer from*
la pulmonía   *pneumonia*
quemarse   *to burn oneself*
el raquitis   *rickets*
rascarse   *to scratch oneself*
sufrir de   *to suffer from*
tener buen apetito   *to have a good appetite*
tener catarro   *to have a cold*
tener diarrea   *to have diarrhea*
tener irritación de la piel   *to have a skin irritation*
toser   *to cough*
vomitar   *to vomit*

Oral practice

Answer the questions using the vocabulary list on childhood ailments and accidents.

1. Cuando el niño elimina demasiado, ¿qué condición tiene?
2. Cuando el niño no puede eliminar, ¿cómo se llama esa condición?
3. Cuando el niño tiene una irritación de la piel, ¿cómo se llama esa condición?
4. ¿Qué enfermedad tiene el niño cuando se pone muy flaco?
5. ¿Qué hace el niño cuando echa comida digerida por la boca?
6. ¿Cómo se llama la condición de la sangre que causa debilidad en una persona?
7. ¿Cómo se llama un catarro muy severo?
8. Cuando el niño come algo que no puede tragar, ¿qué le pasa?
9. ¿Cómo se dice "echarse gases por la boca"?
10. ¿Por qué un niño no debe tocar un cuchillo?

Change the sentences to the imperfect tense following the model.

El bebé tiene catarro hoy.   *The baby has a cold today.*
El bebé tenía catarro todos los días.   *The baby had a cold every day.*

1. El bebé tiene diarrea hoy.
2. El bebé está estreñido hoy.
3. El bebé tiene la piel irritada hoy.
4. El bebé sufre del salpullido hoy.
5. El bebé bebe la leche hoy.
6. El bebé duerme bien hoy.
7. El bebé no elimina bien hoy.
8. El bebé llora mucho hoy.
9. El bebé se enferma hoy.
10. El bebé vomita hoy.

11. El bebé tose mucho hoy.
12. El bebé cólico le molesta a su madre hoy.
13. El bebé no puede dormir hoy.
14. El bebé sufre hoy.
15. El bebé tiene buen apetito hoy.

Change the sentences to the present perfect tense following the model.

La nena tiene impétigo.	*The baby girl has impetigo.*
La nena ha tenido impétigo.	*The baby girl has had impetigo.*

1. Los niños sufren de anemia.
2. Los nenes padecen de pulmonía.
3. El nene sufre de raquitis.
4. La nena se atraganta con el objeto pequeño.
5. Las nenas eructan mucho.
6. El niño se rasca a causa del eczema.
7. La criatura pone el objeto en la boca.
8. La nena se cae de la mesa.
9. El bebé se hace daño con el cuchillo.
10. La niña se quema con el agua hirviente.

Written practice

Translate the sentences into Spanish.

1. Mrs. García's baby has a cold and must stay inside.
2. The mother was worried because her baby had diarrhea.
3. If you clean the baby often, she won't get diaper rash so frequently.
4. The baby is ill and cries a lot.
5. Babies who do not drink enough milk will get rickets.
6. My baby suffers from anemia.
7. Pneumonia is always a very serious illness for a baby.
8. The baby was choking before but she's fine now.
9. The baby fell and got hurt.
10. The baby shouldn't play with sharp objects.

Translate the sentences into English.

1. La madre tiene que cambiarle el pañal al nene.
2. El padre le dio un baño a la criatura.
3. Tengo que ir a la farmacia para comprar la medicina para mi bebé.
4. Tengo una cita con la pediatra la semana que viene.
5. Tengo que esterilizar todos los biberones y los pezones también.
6. Ud. debe probar la leche antes de dársela al bebé.
7. El bebé se enfermó rápidamente.
8. Estoy muy preocupada porque mi bebé tiene pulmonía.

9. La criatura tosía mucho y lloraba toda la noche.
10. Hace dos días que la criatura tiene diarrea.
11. La nena tiene catarro y estornuda mucho.
12. Los bebés sufren de impétigo.
13. La madre no sabía por qué su bebé vomitaba tanto.
14. La criatura enferma se puso muy flaca.
15. Los médicos dicen que su bebé está curado.

Vocabulary

PEDIATRICS / LA PEDIATRÍA

a partir de   *as of, from that date*
asegurar   *to assure*
la buena salud   *good health*
el cereal enriquecido   *enriched cereal*
el cuarto mes   *the fourth month*
un defecto congénito   *a congenital defect*
dentro de   *within*
unos días seguidos   *a few days in a row*
la dislexia   *dyslexia*
durante   *during*
el examen médico   *checkup*

el chequeo   *checkup*
el hierro   *iron*
un impedimento para la lectura   *a reading impediment*
la proteína   *protein*
recomendar   *to recommend*
seco,-a   *dry*
los sólidos   *solids*
tratar   *to treat*
una vez al mes   *once a month*
las vitaminas   *vitamins*
la yema del huevo   *egg yolk*

Conversations

A: Mi bebé y yo vamos a salir del hospital hoy.

B: ¿Cuándo tendrá Ud. que llevarlo al pediatra para su primer chequeo?

A: Dentro de seis semanas. A partir del primer chequeo, tendré que llevarlo una vez al mes durante los seis primeros meses.

B: ¿Por qué es necesario visitar al médico con tanta frecuencia?

A: Para asegurar la buena salud del bebé.

A: Tuve que llamar a la pediatra hoy porque el bebé sufre de irritación de la piel.

B: ¿Qué le dijo la doctora?

A: My baby and I are going to leave the hospital today.

B: When will you have to bring him to the pediatrician for his first checkup?

A: Within six weeks. Starting from the first checkup I will have to bring him once a month for the first six months.

B: Why is it necessary to visit the doctor so frequently?

A: To assure the good health of the child.

A: I had to call the pediatrician today because the baby is suffering from skin rash.

B: What did the doctor tell you?

A: Pues, me dijo que es algo común entre los bebés. Tengo que usar talco y tratar de mantener la piel seca.

B: Entonces, ¿no tiene que llevar al bebé a su consultorio?

A: Solamente si sigue molestándole más de unos días seguidos.

A: ¿Cuándo puedo darle sólidos a mi bebé?

B: Ud. puede darle cereal enriquecido con hierro y vitaminas durante el cuarto mes. También, Ud. puede darle carne colada al mismo tiempo.

A: Me han dicho que es necesario darle la yema del huevo también. ¿Por qué?

B: Porque la yema lleva proteína y muchas vitaminas necesarias para su bebé.

A: ¿Cuántos años tiene su hija?

B: Tiene cinco años.

A: ¿Cuántas veces al año tiene Ud. que llevarla al pediatra?

B: Dos veces al año.

A: ¿Por qué tiene que llevarla hoy?

B: Porque el médico le va a poner unas inyecciones.

A: ¿Por qué está Ud. tan preocupada?

B: Los oficiales de la escuela me han dicho que mi hijo tiene dislexia.

A: ¿Qué es dislexia?

B: Es un impedimento para la lectura. Dicen que es un defecto congénito.

A: ¿Qué va a hacer Ud.?

B: Ellos me han recomendado una escuela especial donde los maestros saben tratar este tipo de problema.

A: Well, she told me that it is something common among babies. I have to use talcum powder and try to keep the skin dry.

B: Then you don't have to take the baby to the doctor's office?

A: Only if it continues to bother him for more than a few days in a row.

A: When can I give solid foods to my baby?

B: You can give him cereal enriched with iron and vitamins during the fourth month. You can also give him strained meat at the same time.

A: I have been told that it is necessary to give him egg yolk also. Why?

B: Because the yolk contains protein and many vitamins necessary for your baby.

A: How old is your daughter?

B: She's five years old.

A: How many times a year do you have to take her to the pediatrician?

B: Two times a year.

A: Why do you have to take her today?

B: Because the doctor is going to give her some injections.

A: Why are you so troubled?

B: The school authorities told me that my son has dyslexia.

A: What is dyslexia?

B: It's a reading impediment. They say that it's a congenital defect.

A: What are you going to do?

B: They have recommended a special school in which the teachers know how to deal with this type of problem.

VOCABULARY

hiperactivo,-a *hyperactive*
tratar de *to try to*
atrasado,-a mentalmente *mentally retarded*

sordo,-a *deaf*
ciego,-a *blind*
el parálisis cerebral *cerebral palsy*
la instrucción *instruction*

estar dispuesto a   *to be prepared to*

enfrentarse con   *to face (a problem, situation)*

confinar en una institución   *to institutionalize*

la terapia   *therapy*

mejorarse   *to improve oneself, to get better*

Role playing

In each of the five sections below you will find three questions dealing with children with special problems. One student asks the questions while the other creates original responses to each question.

1. ¿Es hiperactiva la muchacha?
   ¿Cómo supieron sus padres que es hiperactiva?
   ¿Cómo tratan de ayudarle?

2. ¿Es el niño atrasado mentalmente?
   ¿Están dispuestos sus padres a enfrentarse con el problema?
   ¿Lo van a confinar en una institución?

3. ¿Es sordo el niño?
   ¿Nació sordo?
   ¿Saben los médicos por qué?

4. ¿Es ciega la niña?
   ¿Nació ciega?
   ¿Pueden los médicos operarle los ojos?

5. ¿Tiene parálisis cerebral el niño?
   ¿Recibe instrucción o terapia?
   ¿Se ha mejorado algo?

Cued situation

You are a pediatrician giving instructions to a new mother. Using the vocabulary you have already learned and with the help of the vocabulary below, you must tell her that in her visits it will be necessary to do the following:

A. The child must be immunized against the illnesses and diseases that can occur during childhood. Mention these illnesses and diseases and explain what must be done to prevent them.

B. She must bring the child in for regular physical examinations in order to check the following:

   1. weight
   2. height
   3. general health
   4. development
   5. behavior

C. You will constantly give her advice regarding child care.

VOCABULARY

la bronquitis *bronchitis*	**medir** *measure*
el consejo *advice*	**las paperas** *mumps*
las convulsiones *convulsions*	**pesar** *weigh*
el cuidado *care*	**la poliomielitis** *polio*
el desarrollo *development*	**poner una vacuna** *to vaccinate*
la difteria *diphtheria*	**la rubéola** *rubella*
las enfermedades transmisibles *communicable diseases*	**el sarampión** *measles*
	la tos ferina *whooping cough*
los hábitos *habits*	**la tuberculosis** *tuberculosis*
la infección del oído *ear infection*	**las viruelas locas** *chicken pox*
inmunizar *immunize*	

Dialogue

MÉDICO: Acabo de examinar a su hijo, señora, y está bien de salud. No hay ningún problema.

SEÑORA: Me alegro de eso, doctor. Pero a decir la verdad, tengo un problema que quiero discutir con Ud.

MÉDICO: ¿Qué problema es ése, señora?

SEÑORA: Trato de alimentar bien a mi hijo pero él no quiere comer las comidas buenas.

MÉDICO: ¿Qué come su hijo?

SEÑORA: Toma muchos bocadillos, dulces y refrescos. No le gusta tomar los vegetales ni la leche tampoco.

MÉDICO: Eso es muy malo, señora. Un niño debe acostumbrarse a comer toda clase de comidas. Si no, no va a desarrollarse bien. Debe tomar mucha leche para la proteína y el calcio, los vegetales para las vitaminas y el hierro, y mucha carne también.

SEÑORA: ¿Pero si él no quiere comer?

MÉDICO: Ud. tiene que mantenerse firme, señora. Esto es para la salud de su hijo. No debe mimarle demasiado.

SEÑORA: Sí, doctor, Ud. tiene razón. Trataré de hacer lo que Ud. recomienda.

VOCABULARY

discutir *to discuss*	**toda clase de** *all kinds of*
alimentar *to feed*	**desarrollarse** *to develop*
el bocadillo *snack*	**la proteína** *protein*
los dulces *candy, sweets*	**el calcio** *calcium*
los refrescos *soft drinks*	**el hierro** *iron*
los vegetales *vegetables*	**la carne** *meat*
la leche *milk*	**mantenerse firme** *to be firm*
acostumbrarse a *to get used to*	**mimar** *to spoil*

DOCTOR: I have just examined your son, ma'am, and he is in good health. There isn't any problem.

WOMAN: I'm happy about that, doctor. But to tell the truth, I have a problem which I wish to discuss with you.

DOCTOR: What problem is that, ma'am?

WOMAN: I try to feed my son well but he doesn't want to eat good food.

DOCTOR: What does your son eat?

WOMAN: He eats a lot of snacks, sweets, and soft drinks. He doesn't like to eat vegetables or drink milk either.

DOCTOR: That's very bad, ma'am. A child should get used to eating all kinds of foods. If not, he is not going to develop well. He should drink a lot of milk for protein and calcium, vegetables for vitamins and iron, and a lot of meat also.

WOMAN: But if he doesn't want to eat?

DOCTOR: You must be firm, ma'am. This is for your child's health. You shouldn't spoil him so much.

WOMAN: Yes, doctor, you are right. I shall try to do what you recommend.

QUESTIONS ON DIALOGUE

1. ¿Cuál es el problema de la señora?
2. ¿Qué come su hijo?
3. ¿Qué comidas no le gustan?
4. ¿Qué clase de comidas debe tomar un niño?
5. ¿Para qué se toma la leche? ¿y los vegetales?
6. Según el médico, ¿qué debe hacer la señora?

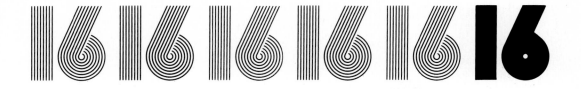

Vocabulary

NUTRITION, DIET, AND FOODS
LA NUTRICIÓN, LA DIETA, Y LAS COMIDAS

EL PAN   BREAD

el pan blanco   *white bread*
el pan de centeno   *rye bread*

el pan de trigo entero   *whole wheat bread*

QUESO Y MANTEQUILLA   CHEESE AND BUTTER

la crema de cacahuete   *peanut butter*
la margarina   *margarine*

el queso crema   *cream cheese*
el requesón   *cottage cheese*

LOS CONDIMENTOS   CONDIMENTS

el aceite   *oil*
el azúcar   *sugar*
las especias   *spices*
la mayonesa   *mayonnaise*

la pimienta   *pepper*
la sacarina   *saccharin*
la sal   *salt*
el vinagre   *vinegar*

EL POSTRE   DESSERT

el bizcocho   *biscuit*
la galleta   *cookie*
la gelatina   *gelatin*
el helado   *ice cream*

el pastel   *pie*
la torta   *cake*
el pudín   *pudding*

LAS BEBIDAS   DRINKS

el agua   *water*
el café   *coffee*
la cerveza   *beer*
el chocolate   *chocolate drink*

el jugo de toronja   *grapefruit juice*
el jugo de china   *orange juice*
el jugo de naranja   *orange juice*
el jugo de tomate   *tomato juice*

la leche *milk*
la limonada *lemonade*
la soda *soda*

el té *tea*
el vino *wine*

LOS HUEVOS   EGGS

los huevos duros *hard-boiled eggs*
los huevos fritos *fried eggs*
los huevos pasados por agua *soft-boiled eggs*

los huevos revueltos *scrambled eggs*
la tortilla *omelette*

EL PESCADO   FISH

las almejas *clams*
el atún *tuna*
los camarones *shrimp*
los cangrejos *crabs*
la langosta *lobster*

los mariscos *shellfish*
las ostras *oysters*
el salmón *salmon*
las sardinas *sardines*

LAS FRUTAS   FRUIT

el albaricoque *apricot*
la cereza *cherry*
la ciruela *plum*
la ciruela pasa *prune*
la fresa *strawberry*
el limón *lemon*

la manzana *apple*
el melocotón *peach*
la naranja *orange*
la pera *pear*
el plátano *banana*
la toronja *grapefruit*

LA CARNE   MEAT

el bistec *steak*
la carne de cordero *lamb*
la carne de puerco *pork*
la carne de res *beef*
la carne de ternera *veal*
la hamburguesa *hamburger*

el jamón *ham*
el pollo *chicken*
el rosbif *roast beef*
la salchicha *sausage*
el tocino *bacon*

LOS VEGETALES Y LAS VERDURAS   VEGETABLES AND GREENS

el apio *celery*
el arroz *rice*
el bróculi *broccoli*
la calabaza *squash*
la cebolla *onion*
la coliflor *cauliflower*
el espárrago *asparagus*
la espinaca *spinach*
el frijol *bean*
el guisante *pea*
la habichuela verde *green bean*

el hongo *mushroom*
la lechuga *lettuce*
el maíz *corn*
las papas asadas *baked potatoes*
las papas fritas *fried potatoes*
el pepino *cucumber*
el pepinillo *pickle*
la remolacha *beet*
el rábano *radish*
el tomate *tomato*
la zanahoria *carrot*

SUPPLEMENTARY VOCABULARY ON FOODS

los alimentos *food*
almorzar *to lunch*
tomar el almuerzo *to have lunch*
beneficioso,-a *beneficial*
la cantidad *quantity*
cenar *to dine*
la comida *meal*
la contaminación *contamination*
desayunarse *to breakfast*
tomar el desayuno *to have breakfast*

una dieta baja en calorías *a low-calorie diet*
una dieta balanceada *a balanced diet*
evitar *to avoid*
la grasa *fat*
indigestible *indigestible*
limitado,-a *limited*
los minerales *minerals*
la resistencia *resistance, stamina, endurance*
tomar *to drink, to eat*

Written practice

In the questions below you are required to prepare several types of diets. Use the above vocabulary lists to form these diet plans.

1. ¿Qué se puede tomar para el desayuno si uno está siguiendo una dieta balanceada? ¿para el almuerzo? ¿para la cena?
2. ¿Qué alimentos se deben evitar si uno está siguiendo una dieta baja en calorías?
3. ¿Puede Ud. recomendar un plan diario para una persona que debe seguir una dieta baja en sal? ¿en colesterol? ¿sin alimentos indigestibles?
4. ¿Qué alimentos no debe comer uno si tiene diabetis?
5. ¿Qué alimentos no debe comer uno si tiene úlceras? ¿gastritis?

Oral practice

Change the sentences to direct commands following the model.

Ud. tiene que tomar mucha agua.   *You must drink a lot of water.*
Tome Ud. mucha agua.   *Drink a lot of water.*

1. Ud. tiene que comer mucha carne.
2. Ud. tiene que preparar la comida.
3. Ud. tiene que tomar vitaminas.
4. Ud. tiene que beber mucha leche.
5. Ud. tiene que tomar mucho jugo.
6. Ud. tiene que comprar mucho queso.
7. Ud. tiene que cocinar comidas ricas en minerales.
8. Ud. tiene que seguir una dieta balanceada.
9. Ud. tiene que comer muchas frutas.
10. Ud. tiene que perder mucho peso.
11. Ud. tiene que evitar el uso de especias.
12. Ud. tiene que usar las especias con cuidado.

13. Ud. tiene que aprender a cocinar.
14. Ud. tiene que lavar los platos.
15. Ud. tiene que pesarse.

Answer the questions with complete sentences.

1. ¿Prefiere Ud. beber jugo de china o jugo de tomate?
2. ¿Qué le gusta tomar más, el café o el té?
3. ¿Va Ud. a comprar el pan blanco o el pan de centeno?
4. ¿Usa Ud. la sal y la pimienta?
5. ¿Usa Ud. la sacarina o el azúcar?
6. ¿Necesita Ud. comprar el queso crema o el requesón?
7. ¿Tiene Ud. que comprar peras o plátanos?
8. ¿Va Ud. a comprar fresas o cerezas?
9. ¿Va Ud. a preparar pastel de limón o pastel de manzanas?
10. ¿Prefiere Ud. los huevos duros o los huevos pasados por agua?
11. ¿Qué desea Ud. más, los camarones o la langosta?
12. ¿Qué tiene Ud. que evitar, la carne frita o la carne asada?
13. ¿Qué toma Ud. para la cena, el jamón o el arroz con pollo?
14. ¿Qué va Ud. a echar en la sopa, el apio o los guisantes?
15. ¿Qué quiere Ud. comer con la cena, la coliflor o el bróculi?

Change the sentences from the present to the preterite tense.

1. El médico recomienda una dieta especial.
2. Tomo el desayuno a las siete.
3. La mujer compra los vegetales.
4. El hombre sigue una dieta para los diabéticos.
5. Usamos muchas especias en la comida.
6. La muchacha toma el postre.
7. Los pacientes beben la leche.
8. Pierdo mucho peso.
9. El joven toma el almuerzo al mediodía.
10. Las muchachas lavan los platos y limpian la cocina.

Change the sentences from the present to the imperfect tense.

1. Necesito seguir una dieta estricta.
2. El médico prepara una dieta especial para el diabético.
3. La muchacha bebe el jugo de china.
4. El paciente come los vegetales.
5. La joven sigue una dieta sin sal.
6. Es una dieta baja en colesterol.
7. No usamos sal.
8. La paciente evita el uso de especias.
9. Vamos a comprar el rosbif y la carne de ternera.
10. El hombre tiene problemas gastrointestinales.

Conversation

A: ¿Qué me recomienda Ud., doctor? Me siento tan débil.

A: What do you recommend, doctor? I feel so weak.

B: Ud. en realidad no está enfermo. Es que no come bien. Le recomiendo una dieta balanceada.

B: In reality, you aren't ill. It's that you don't eat well. I recommend a balanced diet.

A: Pero yo como bien.

A: But I eat well.

B: Ud. no come comidas buenas. Tiene que comer comidas ricas en proteína y vitaminas.

B: You don't eat good food. You have to eat foods which are rich in protein and vitamins.

A: Pero muchas veces no tengo el tiempo para comer, y además, la comida es cara.

A: But often I don't have the time to eat, and besides, food is expensive.

B: Entonces, le recomiendo un suplemento de vitaminas en forma de una pastilla.

B: Well then, I'm recommending a vitamin supplement for you in the form of a pill.

Written practice

Translate the sentences into English.

1. Los que tienen catarro deben tomar muchos líquidos.
2. El pescado es una comida muy buena porque lleva mucha proteína y poca grasa.
3. Las especias siempre deben usarse con cuidado, especialmente para los que tienen problemas digestivos.
4. Ud. debe tomar el té en vez del café.
5. El señor García dice que no le gustan las verduras.
6. La señora dice que a menudo comía antes de acostarse.
7. Es importante cocinar bien la carne de puerco para evitar la contaminación.
8. El médico me dijo que mi hijo tiene poca resistencia a las enfermedades porque no come bastante.
9. El médico recomendó una dieta muy estricta para la paciente en el cuarto 259.
10. El médico me dijo que tengo gastritis.

Translate the sentences into Spanish.

1. Spinach is a vegetable that contains iron.
2. People who wish to lose weight should eat low-calorie foods.
3. You must prepare foods that are rich in vitamins and minerals.
4. I have to go shopping because I need carrots, celery, onions, and squash.
5. She used to use a lot of spices in her meals.
6. Because I have ulcers, I have to follow a special diet.
7. She needed to buy fresh fruit and vegetables.
8. Can I eat lamb, pork, and beef?
9. It is necessary to eat foods that are low in cholesterol.
10. The patient couldn't eat his dessert.

Reading

La nutrición es uno de los factores más importantes para el bienestar físico y emocional de una persona. Para evitar las enfermedades se tiene que seguir una dieta balanceada. Además, hay muchas dietas especiales que ayudan a curar ciertas enfermedades y malestares. Si uno piensa especializarse en cualquier profesión médica, tiene que familiarizarse con la nutrición, la dieta y los alimentos básicos. Si tiene el conocimiento adecuado, podrá informar al paciente en cuanto a lo que debe y no debe comer.

Si uno quiere seguir una dieta balanceada, debe comer alimentos ricos en proteína como la carne, la leche, los cereales, el queso, y los huevos. También debe comer vegetales ricos en vitaminas como la lechuga, la espinaca, los guisantes, el maíz, y el apio.

Hay también las dietas especiales para los que sufren de enfermedades específicas. Por ejemplo, una dieta blanda, con poca acidez y pocos alimentos indigestibles es apropiada para las enfermedades gastrointestinales. Para los que tienen la presión alta, se recomienda una dieta sin sal. En todo caso, el que tiene una enfermedad debe seguir una dieta especial. El médico o el especialista es responsable de recomendarle al paciente la dieta más beneficiosa para su salud.

VOCABULARY

el bienestar *well-being*
físico,-a *physical*
emocional *emotional*
evitar *to avoid*
el malestar *ailment*
pensar + infinitive *to intend to*
especializarse en *to specialize in*

familiarizarse con *to familiarize oneself with*
el conocimiento *knowledge*
adecuado,-a *adequate*
en cuanto a *as to, concerning*
específico,-a *specific*
la acidez *acidity*
responsable *responsible*

QUESTIONS ON READING

1. ¿Qué hay que hacer para evitar las enfermedades?
2. ¿Por qué es necesario familiarizarse con la nutrición?
3. ¿Qué clase de alimentos se deben evitar si uno está siguiendo una dieta blanda?
4. ¿Para qué enfermedades es apropiada una dieta blanda?
5. ¿Qué dieta se debe seguir si se tiene la presión alta?
6. ¿Quién es el responsable de recomendar una dieta al paciente?

Dialogue

PACIENTE: Doctora, muchas veces tengo dolor del estómago.
DOCTORA: ¿Cuándo son más fuertes los dolores?
PACIENTE: Me duele más al despertarme por la mañana y antes de comer.
DOCTORA: ¿Qué clase de dolor es?
PACIENTE: Pues, es una sensación agria, como de náuseas.

DOCTORA: ¿Es Ud. un hombre nervioso?

PACIENTE: Sí, por lo general. Tengo muchos problemas en mi familia y en mi trabajo y me pongo nervioso a menudo.

DOCTORA: Creo que lo que Ud. tiene es un caso de gastritis. Le voy a mandar al laboratorio para una radiografía del sistema digestivo. Pero ahora le voy a dar una dieta que tiene que seguir.

PACIENTE: ¿Qué clase de dieta es?

DOCTORA: Es una dieta de comidas blandas para neutralizar el ácido del estómago. No debe tomar café, bebidas alcohólicas, comidas grasosas o fritas o difíciles de digerir, y no debe fumar cigarrillos. Por otra parte, debe tomar mucha leche, pan blanco, y sopas blandas.

PACIENTE: Es una dieta muy estricta. ¿Por cuánto tiempo tengo que seguirla?

DOCTORA: Si Ud. la sigue al pie de la letra, se curará dentro de seis semanas.

PACIENTE: ¿Puede Ud. recetarme algo?

DOCTORA: Ud. debe tomar un antiácido pero para eso no se necesita una receta. Se puede comprar en cualquier farmacia.

PACIENTE: ¿Hay algo más que debo hacer?

DOCTORA: Sí. Ud. debe tratar de quedarse tranquilo. No se ponga tan nervioso. Ahora es cuestión de la salud.

VOCABULARY

agrio,-a *sour*
ponerse + adjective *to become*
blando,-a *bland*
neutralizar *neutralize*
el ácido *acid, acidity*
grasoso,-a *greasy*

digerir *digest*
al pie de la letra *verbatim*
el antiácido *antacid*
cualquier *any*
una cuestión *issue, matter, question*

PATIENT: Doctor, I often get pains in my stomach.

DOCTOR: When are the pains most severe?

PATIENT: It hurts the most when I wake up in the morning and before I eat.

DOCTOR: What type of pain is it?

PATIENT: Well, it's a sour feeling, like nausea.

DOCTOR: Are you a nervous man?

PATIENT: Yes, generally. I have many problems with my family and with my job, and I often become nervous.

DOCTOR: I believe that what you have is a case of gastritis. I'm going to send you to the lab for an X-ray of your digestive tract. But for now I am going to give you a diet that you must follow.

PATIENT: What kind of diet is it?

DOCTOR: It is a diet of bland foods to neutralize the acidity in your stomach. You shouldn't have coffee, greasy or fried foods, foods that are difficult to digest, and you must not smoke cigarettes. On the other hand, you should have plenty of milk, white bread, and bland soups.

PATIENT: It's a very strict diet. How long must I follow it?

DOCTOR: If you follow it to the letter, you will be cured within six weeks.

PATIENT: Can you prescribe something for me?

DOCTOR: You should take an antacid but you don't need a prescription for that. You can buy it in any drugstore.

PATIENT: Is there anything else I should do?

DOCTOR: Yes, You should try to stay calm. Don't get so nervous. Now it's a question of your health.

QUESTIONS ON DIALOGUE

1. ¿Dónde tiene dolor el paciente?
2. ¿Cuándo son más fuertes estos dolores?
3. ¿Cómo es el dolor?
4. ¿Es el paciente un hombre nervioso? ¿Por qué?
5. Según la doctora, ¿qué tiene el paciente?
6. ¿A dónde le va a mandar la doctora?
7. ¿Qué clase de dieta le da la doctora al paciente?
8. ¿Qué no debe tomar el paciente?
9. ¿Qué comidas le recomienda la doctora?
10. ¿Por cuánto tiempo tiene el paciente que seguir la dieta?
11. ¿Qué medicina va a tomar el hombre?
12. Por fin, ¿qué le recomienda la doctora al paciente?

ANALYSIS OF DIALOGUE

1. ¿Cree Ud. que la doctora tiene razón al recomendar una dieta antes de tener los resultados de la radiografía?
2. ¿Es una dieta blanda la mejor para problemas gastrointestinales?
3. ¿Qué otras comidas no se deben tomar en una dieta blanda? ¿Qué otras comidas son beneficiosas?

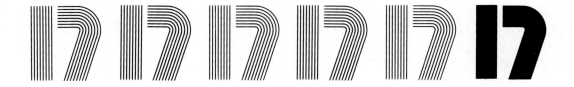

Vocabulary

THE NURSE, THE PATIENT, AND THE HOSPITAL

LA ENFERMERA, EL PACIENTE, Y EL HOSPITAL

LA ENFERMERA, EL ENFERMERO   THE NURSE

cambiar la venda   *to change the bandage*

cambiar el vendaje   *to change the dressing*

consultar con el médico   *to consult with the doctor*

dar de comer   *to feed*

dar la medicina   *to give the medicine*

dar un baño   *to give a bath*

examinar el vendaje   *to examine the dressing*

hacer la cama   *to make the bed*

insertar el catéter, la sonda, el tubo   *to insert the catheter*

poner el aire acondicionado   *to put on the air conditioning*

poner una enema, una ayuda, un lavado, una lavativa   *to give an enema*

poner una inyección   *to give an injection*

registrar el pulso   *to take the pulse*

tomar la presión   *to take the blood pressure*

tomar la temperatura   *to take the temperature*

EL/LA PACIENTE   THE PATIENT

la almohada   *pillow*

la autorización para la cirugía   *authorization for surgery*

el bacín   *bedpan*

el baño   *bath*

la bata   *bathrobe*

la cama   *bed*

el cepillo de dientes   *toothbrush*

el cuarto   *room*

el cuarto doble, múltiple, privado   *double room, ward, private*

fumar   *to smoke*

el jabón   *soap*

la manta   *blanket*

la operación   *operation*

el permiso   *permission*

las pijamas *pajamas*
sentirse mareado,-a *to feel dizzy*
sentirse molesto,-a *to feel bothered*
tener dolor *to be in pain*

tener náuseas *to be nauseous*
la toalla *towel*
las zapatillas *slippers*

Oral practice

In the following exercise you are required to respond to a variety of specific patient complaints and questions. You must create questions or responses which correspond to each of the five cues given for each of the five sections. For example:

Tengo dolor
• señalar
Señáleme Ud. donde le duele.

I am in pain
• *to show*
Show me where it hurts.

1. No puedo dormir.
   • estar nervioso   • tener miedo   • los problemas   • la familia   • tener dolor

2. No quiero tomar el desayuno.
   • gustar   • la comida   • el apetito   • la digestión   • la medicina

3. No he podido eliminar.
   • el médico   • examinar   • aliviar   • ayudar   • poner una enema

4. ¿Por qué me molesta Ud. tanto?
   • tener que   • lavar   • hacer la cama   • cambiar el vendaje   • dar un baño

5. ¿Qué me va a hacer Ud.?
   • poner una inyección   • tomar la temperatura   • registrar el pulso   • lavar
   • dar el medicamento

6. Me duele la herida.
   • tipo de dolor   • sentirse débil   • limpiar   • cambiar el vendaje
   • el medicamento

7. ¿Qué me hace Ud.?
   • insertar un catéter   • poner una inyección intravenosa   • calmarse
   • nervioso   • quejarse

8. Tengo que orinar.
   • el bacín   • tocar el timbre   • terminar   • sentirse mejor   • beber

9. No me gusta este cuarto doble.
   • quejarse   • el otro paciente   • un cuarto privado   • ocupado   • el ruido

10. Mi hijo me llevó mis pijamas.
    • la bata   • el cepillo de dientes   • las zapatillas   • unas revistas
    • el periódico

11. ¿Cuándo me van a operar?
    • necesitar la autorización   • el permiso   • firmar   • la cirugía   • grave

12. No me siento cómodo.
    - la almohada   • la manta   • el aire acondicionado
    - encender (apagar) la luz   • el calor

13. Tengo náuseas.
    - la vasija de vómito   • el lavabo   • la medicina   • la comida
    - llamar al médico

14. No me gusta la comida del hospital.
    - tener que   • la dieta   • las órdenes del médico   • los vegetales
    - sentirse mejor

15. ¿Me va a bañar ahora?
    - el agua caliente   • el jabón   • la toalla   • limpiar   • sucio

Conversations

A: El médico dice que su mamá necesitará una operación para quitarle el quiste.

A: The doctor says that your mother will need an operation in order to remove the cyst.

B: Creía que su caso no era tan grave.

B: I thought that her case wasn't so serious.

A: No es muy grave. Es una operación muy fácil y no hay peligro.

A: It isn't very serious. It's a simple operation and there is no danger.

B: ¿Cuándo le van a operar?

B: When are they going to operate?

A: Le van a operar tan pronto como posible. Quizás, el día pasado mañana.

A: They are going to operate as soon as possible. Perhaps the day after tomorrow.

B: ¿Me informará Ud. de todo?

B: Will you keep me informed of everything?

A: Sí, por supuesto.

A: Yes, of course.

A: Señorita, tengo mucho calor. Creo que tengo calentura.

A: Miss, I'm very hot. I think I have a fever.

B: Voy a tomarle la temperatura. No, Ud. no tiene calentura.

B: I am going to take your temperature. No, you don't have a fever.

A: Entonces, ¿por qué tengo tanto calor?

A: Then why am I so hot?

B: Ud. debe de estar nervioso. Voy a darle un calmante.

B: You must be nervous. I'm going to give you a sedative.

A: ¿Cómo se llama Ud.?

A: What is your name?

B: Me llamo Ángel Vásquez.

B: My name is Ángel Vásquez.

A: ¿Cómo se lastimó la cabeza?

A: How did you hurt your head?

B: Me caí escalera abajo.

B: I fell down the stairs.

A: ¿Cuándo ocurrió esto?

A: When did this happen?

B: Ocurrió hace un par de horas.

B: It happened a couple of hours ago.

Written practice

Translate the sentences into English.

1. No se permite fumar en el hospital.
2. El paciente prefiere un cuarto privado.
3. ¿Por qué necesita el médico una autorización para la cirugía?
4. Tengo que examinar el vendaje.
5. Es necesario ponerle una enema al paciente.
6. Señorita, me siento mareado y tengo náuseas.
7. Debo hacer las camas en el cuarto doce.
8. ¿Quiere Ud. ponerse la bata ahora, señora Menéndez?
9. La enfermera me da la medicina a las doce del mediodía.
10. ¿Necesita Ud. usar el bacín?

Translate the sentences into Spanish.

1. I am going to take your pulse now.
2. When can I leave the hospital?
3. I must give you an injection.
4. Would you please turn on the air conditioning?
5. The nurse consulted with the doctor this morning.
6. The nurse is going to change my bandage soon.
7. You must give the patient the medicine every six hours.
8. First I am going to take your temperature and then, your pressure.
9. I must give a bath to the patient in room thirty-six.
10. If you feel dizzy, you should lie down.

Reading

Los deberes de los enfermeros en el hospital son muy variados. Una de sus funciones más importantes es cuidar de las necesidades físicas del paciente. Por ejemplo, el enfermero o la enfermera tiene que darle de comer, tomarle la temperatura y la presión, registrarle el pulso y bañarle. Tiene otras responsabilidades también. Debe ponerle las inyecciones necesarias al paciente y darle el medicamento recetado por el médico. Además, la enfermera o el enfermero debe tener la habilidad para comprender los diagnósticos y los pronósticos y debe poder ejercer todas las funciones del médico, si éste no está presente.

Muchas veces las responsabilidades de los enfermeros dependen de la especialización escojida. Si están en la sala de partos ayudan a la madre en la labor y al médico también. Si están en la sala de emergencias tienen que estar preparados para cualquier caso. En la sala de operaciones la enfermera o el enfermero ayuda al médico y tiene que estar familiarizado con todos los instrumentos y aparatos allí.

La función más importante de todas para los enfermeros realmente no tiene que ver con los aspectos técnicos de la medicina. La enfermera o el enfermero es el vínculo entre el paciente y el hospital. Ellos le hacen sentirse cómodo en un ambiente extraño e incomprensible como es la institución del hospital. Esto es porque tienen probablemente más contacto personal con el paciente que cualquier otra persona en el hospital.

VOCABULARY

los deberes *duties*	**ejercer** *to carry out*
variado,-a *varied*	**la especialización** *specialization*
la función *function*	**escojido,-a** *chosen*
la responsabilidad *responsibility*	**tener que ver con** *to have to do with*
recetado,-a por *prescribed by*	**el vínculo** *link*
la habilidad *ability*	**el ambiente** *atmosphere*
el pronóstico *prognosis*	

QUESTIONS ON READING

1. ¿Cuáles son algunos de los deberes de los enfermeros en el hospital?
2. ¿Cómo se determinan las responsabilidades de los enfermeros?
3. ¿Qué hacen los enfermeros que están asignados a (*assigned to*) la sala de partos? ¿a la sala de operaciones?
4. ¿Cuál es la función más importante de la enfermera o el enfermero?

QUESTIONS FOR DISCUSSION

1. ¿Cuáles son algunas otras responsabilidades de los enfermeros?
2. ¿Cómo se distinguen sus responsabilidades de las del médico? ¿Qué deberes tienen en común?
3. ¿Cree Ud. que los enfermeros están en la mejor posición para tener un contacto personal con el paciente?

Dialogue

ENFERMERA: ¿Cómo se siente Ud. hoy, señor Moreno?

PACIENTE: Estoy muy débil.

ENFERMERA: Eso es de esperar. Ud. es muy anciano y acaba de tener una operación muy importante. ¿Siente Ud. náuseas?

PACIENTE: No. Pero estoy un poco mareado.

ENFERMERA: Eso no es un problema. Después de tomar este medicamento Ud. se sentirá mejor. ¿Necesita Ud. el bacín?

PACIENTE: No, no lo necesito.

ENFERMERA: Muy bien. Ahora voy a tomarle la temperatura y la presión y registrarle el pulso.

PACIENTE: ¿Por qué me tiene que hacer estas cosas tantas veces? ¿No pueden Uds. dejarme en paz?

ENFERMERA: Hay que hacer estas cosas si quiere salir de aquí y volver pronto a casa.

PACIENTE: A propósito, ¿cuándo podré volver a casa?

ENFERMERA: El doctor Weston dice que la operación salió bien y que Ud. podrá volver a casa dentro de una semana.

PACIENTE: ¡Gracias a Dios!

ENFERMERA: Pero Ud. tendrá que seguir una dieta muy estricta.

PACIENTE: Las dietas son una molestia.

ENFERMERA: Sí, pero hay que seguirlas . . .

PACIENTE: ¡Ah! ¡Aquí viene mi hija!

HIJA: Hola papacito, ¿qué tal?

PACIENTE: Estoy bien, pero me molesta este hospital porque tiene tantas reglas y dietas y pruebas.

ENFERMERA: Acabo de explicarle a su papá la importancia de seguir la dieta recomendada por el médico.

HIJA: Sí, por supuesto, la dieta es muy importante. Papá va a quedarse conmigo un par de meses y yo le cuidaré bien.

ENFERMERA: Eso es mucho mejor. Yo sé que de esta manera su papá quedará bien curado. Con su permiso, tengo que ver a otro paciente ahora. Hasta luego.

HIJA: Muchas gracias, señorita. Hasta luego.

VOCABULARY

anciano,-a *elderly*

acabar de *to have just*

mareado,-a *dizzy*

dejarle (a uno) en paz *to leave (one) in peace*

volver *to return*

pronto *soon*

salir bien *to turn out well*

¡Gracias a Dios! *Thank God!*

una molestia *a bother*

hola *hello*

papacito *daddy*

¿Qué tal? *How are you?*

las reglas *rules*

un par *a pair, a couple*

con su permiso *excuse me*

NURSE: How do you feel today, Mr. Moreno?

PATIENT: I'm very weak.

NURSE: That is to be expected. You are very old and you have just had a very important operation. Do you feel nauseous?

PATIENT: No, but I'm a little dizzy.

NURSE: That's not a problem. After you take this medication you will feel better. Do you need the bedpan?

PATIENT: No, I don't need it.

NURSE: Very well. Now I am going to take your temperature, blood pressure, and pulse.

PATIENT: Why do you have to do these things to me so many times? Can't you leave me in peace?

NURSE: These things must be done if you are to leave here and return home soon.

PATIENT: By the way, when will I be able to return home?

NURSE:	Doctor Weston says that the operation was a success and that you will be able to return home within a week.
PATIENT:	Thank God!
NURSE:	But you will have to follow a very strict diet.
PATIENT:	Diets are a bother.
NURSE:	Yes, but you must follow them.
PATIENT:	Ah! Here comes my daughter!
DAUGHTER:	Hello, Daddy, how are you?
PATIENT:	I'm fine but this hospital bothers me because it has so many rules, diets, and tests.
NURSE:	I have just explained to your father the importance of following the diet recommended by the physician.
DAUGHTER:	Yes, of course, the diet is very important. Father is going to stay with me for a couple of months and I will take good care of him.
NURSE:	That is much better. I'm sure that if that's the case your father is going to get well. Excuse me, I have to see another patient now. See you later.
DAUGHTER:	Thank you very much, miss. Goodbye.

QUESTIONS ON DIALOGUE

1. ¿Cómo se siente el señor Moreno?
2. ¿Siente náuseas? ¿Se siente mareado?
3. ¿Qué se hará para sentirse mejor?
4. ¿Necesita él el bacín?
5. ¿De qué se queja el señor Moreno?
6. ¿Cuándo podrá volver a casa?
7. ¿Cómo responde la enfermera a sus quejas?
8. ¿Qué tendrá que hacer el señor Moreno al volver a casa?
9. ¿Qué piensa el señor Moreno de las dietas?
10. ¿Con quién se va a quedar el señor Moreno?

ANALYSIS OF DIALOGUE

1. ¿Por qué se queja tanto el señor Moreno?
2. ¿Cree Ud. que la enfermera ha respondido bien a las preguntas del anciano?
3. En este diálogo, la enfermera se dirige a la hija del enfermo. ¿Es importante tener buenas relaciones con los familiares y parientes de un enfermo? ¿Por qué?

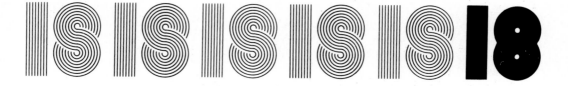

Tests and Procedures
Pruebas y Procedimientos

Vocabulary

ANESTHESIOLOGY/LA ANESTESIOLOGÍA

la alergia *allergy*
la anestesia *anesthesia*
el anestesiólogo *anesthesiologist*
el anestético *anesthetic*
el asma *asthma*
la cirugía *surgery*
tener catarro *to have a cold*

la fiebre de heno *hay fever*
hacer una pregunta *to ask a question*
operar *to operate*
preocuparse *to worry*
la sala de recuperación *recovery room*
la úlcera *ulcer*

Dialogue

ANESTESIÓLOGO: Buenos días, señora García. Yo soy el anestesiólogo, el doctor Perkins. Como Ud. ya sabe, le van a operar la úlcera mañana. Yo le voy a dar el anestético.

PACIENTE: ¿A qué hora me van a operar?

ANESTESIÓLOGO: A las nueve de la mañana. No se preocupe tanto. Todo va bien. Por ahora, tengo que hacerle unas preguntas importantes. ¿Está bien?

PACIENTE: Sí, cómo no, doctor.

ANESTESIÓLOGO: Entonces, primero, ¿sufre Ud. de asma?

PACIENTE: No, no sufro de asma.

ANESTESIÓLOGO: ¿Sufre Ud. de fiebre de heno o de alergias?

PACIENTE:	No, no sufro de ninguna alergia.
ANESTESIÓLOGO:	¿Sufre Ud. del corazón, de los pulmones, o de los riñones?
PACIENTE:	Creo que no.
ANESTESIÓLOGO:	¿Sufre Ud. de la presión alta o de la presión baja?
PACIENTE:	No, doctor.
ANESTESIÓLOGO:	¿Tiene Ud. catarro? ¿Le duele la garganta?
PACIENTE:	No, no tengo catarro y no me duele la garganta.
ANESTESIÓLOGO:	¿Tiene Ud. tos?
PACIENTE:	Tengo un poco de tos pero creo que es de los nervios.
ANESTESIÓLOGO:	Entonces, eso es todo. No se preocupe Ud. Le vamos a poner una inyección en el brazo y Ud. va a dormir. Después de la cirugía, le van a llevar a la sala de recuperación. Hasta mañana, señora.
PACIENTE:	Hasta mañana, doctor.

ANESTHESIOLOGIST:	Good morning, Mrs. García. I am the anesthesiologist, Dr. Perkins. As you already know, they are going to operate on your ulcer tomorrow. I am going to give you the anesthetic.
PATIENT:	What time are they going to operate on me?
ANESTHESIOLOGIST:	At nine in the morning. Don't worry so much. Everything is going fine. For now, I have to ask you some important questions. Is that all right?
PATIENT:	Yes, of course, doctor.
ANESTHESIOLOGIST:	Well then, first, do you suffer from asthma?
PATIENT:	No, I don't suffer from asthma.
ANESTHESIOLOGIST:	Do you suffer from hay fever or from allergies?
PATIENT:	No, I don't suffer from any allergy.
ANESTHESIOLOGIST:	Do you have problems with your heart, your lungs, or your kidneys?
PATIENT:	I don't think so.
ANESTHESIOLOGIST:	Do you suffer from high or low blood pressure?
PATIENT:	No, doctor.
ANESTHESIOLOGIST:	Do you have a cold? Does your throat hurt?
PATIENT:	No, I don't have a cold and my throat doesn't hurt.
ANESTHESIOLOGIST:	Do you have a cough?
PATIENT:	I have a little cough but I think that it's from nerves.
ANESTHESIOLOGIST:	Then, that is all. Don't worry. We are going to give you an injection in your arm and you will go to sleep. After surgery, they are going to take you to the recovery room. Until tomorrow, ma'am.
PATIENT:	Until tomorrow, doctor.

QUESTIONS ON DIALOGUE

1. ¿Quién es el doctor Perkins?
2. ¿Cuándo le van a operar a la señora García?
3. ¿Qué le van a operar a la señora?
4. ¿Sufre la señora del corazón, de los pulmones o de los riñones?

5. ¿Tiene tos la señora?
6. ¿En qué parte del cuerpo le van a poner la inyección?
7. ¿A dónde van a llevar a la señora después de la operación?

Written practice

Translate the sentences into Spanish (**Ud.** commands).

1. Lie down on your stomach.
2. Lie down on your back, please.
3. Lie down on your left side.
4. Sit up.
5. Don't move.
6. Breathe deeply.
7. Bend your knees.
8. Bring your knees to your chest.
9. Turn over.
10. Count to ten, slowly.

Vocabulary

X-RAYS / LAS RADIOGRAFÍAS

durar   *to last*
enfrente de   *in front of*
hacer una radiografía   *to take an X-ray*
indicar   *to indicate, show, point out*

la máquina   *the machine*
pararse   *to stand*
la prueba   *test*
quitarse   *to take off*

Conversation

TÉCNICO: Le voy a hacer una radiografía del pecho.

PACIENTE: ¿Qué indicará la radiografía?

TÉCNICO: Indicará si Ud. tiene una enfermedad de los pulmones como la tuberculosis o la pleuresía.

PACIENTE: ¿Qué tengo que hacer?

TÉCNICO: Tiene que quitarse la camisa y pararse enfrente de esta máquina.

PACIENTE: ¿Durará mucho tiempo?

TÉCNICO: No. Sólo durará unos momentos.

PACIENTE: ¿Me va a doler?

TÉCNICO: No. Ud. no va a sentir nada.

TECHNICIAN: I am going to give you a chest X-ray.

PATIENT: What will this X-ray show?

TECHNICIAN: It will show if you have a chest disease like tuberculosis or pleurisy.

PATIENT: What must I do?

TECHNICIAN: You must take off your shirt and stand in front of this machine.

PATIENT: Will it take a long time?

TECHNICIAN: No, it will only take a few moments.

PATIENT: Will it hurt me?

TECHNICIAN: No, you won't feel anything.

QUESTIONS ON CONVERSATION

1. ¿Qué va a hacer el técnico al paciente?
2. ¿Qué indicará la prueba?
3. ¿Qué tiene que hacer el paciente?
4. ¿Cuánto tiempo durará la prueba?
5. ¿Le va a doler al paciente?

Written practice

Translate the sentences into Spanish.

1. I am going to X-ray your arm.
2. The X-ray will show if it is broken.
3. The patient must take off his shirt.
4. He will have to stand in front of the machine.
5. This test will not take long.

SUPPLEMENTARY VOCABULARY ON X-RAYS

apretar   *to press*
el calambre   *cramp*
estar estreñido   *to be constipated*
saber mal   *to taste bad*

el sistema digestivo   *digestive system*
el sulfato de bario   *barium sulfate*
tratar de   *to try to*
el tumor   *tumor*

Conversation

MÉDICO: Tenemos que hacerle unas radiografías. Vamos a tratar de determinar si tiene úlceras o un tumor en el sistema digestivo.

DOCTOR: We have to take some X-rays. We are going to try to determine if you have ulcers or a tumor in your digestive system.

PACIENTE: ¿Qué me van a hacer?

PATIENT: What are you going to do to me?

MÉDICO: Tiene que tomar este líquido. Se llama el sulfato de bario. Sabe mal. Tengo que apretarle el estómago.

DOCTOR: You have to drink this liquid. It is called barium sulfate. It tastes bad. I have to press your stomach.

PACIENTE: ¿Me va a doler mucho?

PATIENT: Will it hurt much?

MÉDICO: Posiblemente tendrá calambres y estará estreñido.

DOCTOR: You might have cramps and be constipated.

PACIENTE: ¿Va a durar mucho?

PATIENT: Will it last long?

MÉDICO: Durará unos cuarenta y cinco minutos más o menos.

DOCTOR: It will last around forty-five minutes more or less.

QUESTIONS ON CONVERSATION

1. ¿Qué le van a hacer al paciente?
2. ¿Qué piensan determinar los médicos?
3. ¿Qué tiene que tomar el paciente?
4. ¿Habrá efectos secundarios?
5. ¿Durará mucho?

Written practice

Translate the sentences into Spanish.

1. This liquid tastes bad.
2. You have a tumor in your digestive tract.
3. I have very strong cramps.
4. It hurts when you press down on my stomach.
5. Are you going to remove the tumor?

Conversation

X-RAYS: LOWER DIGESTIVE TRACT

LAS RADIOGRAFÍAS: LA PARTE INFERIOR DEL SISTEMA DIGESTIVO

MÉDICO: Vamos a hacerle unas radiografías, pero primero, tenemos que ponerle una enema. Llevará una solución de sulfato de bario.

DOCTOR: We are going to take some X-rays, but first, we have to give you an enema. It will contain a barium sulfate solution.

PACIENTE: ¿Por qué me tiene que hacer esto?

PATIENT: Why do you have to give me this?

MÉDICO: Tenemos que averiguar si tiene úlceras en la parte inferior del sistema digestivo.

DOCTOR: We have to find out if you have ulcers in your lower digestive tract.

PACIENTE: ¿Habrá efectos secundarios?

PATIENT: Will there be side effects?

MÉDICO: Posiblemente tendrá calambres.

DOCTOR: Possibly you will have cramps.

QUESTIONS ON CONVERSATION

1. ¿Qué llevará la enema?
2. ¿Por qué van a hacer las radiografías?
3. ¿Va a sufrir efectos secundarios el paciente?

Written Practice

Translate the sentences into Spanish.

1. My doctor thinks I have an ulcer.
2. He is going to give me an enema.
3. I'm nervous because there will be side effects.
4. They are going to operate on my ulcer.
5. We have to take the X-rays now.

Vocabulary

X-RAYS: GALLBLADDER
LAS RADIOGRAFÍAS: LA VESÍCULA BILIAR

el catéter   *catheter*
el conducto biliar   *bile duct*
funcionar mal   *to malfunction*
insertar   *to insert*
inyectar   *to inject*
molestar   *to bother*

las piedras biliares   *gallstones*
el riesgo   *risk*
la tinta   *dye*
el tubo   *tube*
la vesícula biliar   *gallbladder*

Conversation

MÉDICO: Vamos a hacerle unas radiografías de la vesícula biliar.

DOCTOR: We are going to do some X-rays of your gallbladder.

PACIENTE: ¿Por qué me van a hacer esto?

PATIENT: Why are you going to do this to me?

MÉDICO: Creemos que este órgano funciona mal. Además queremos determinar si tiene piedras biliares.

DOCTOR: We believe that this organ is malfunctioning. In addition, we want to determine if you have gallstones.

PACIENTE: ¿Cómo van a hacer la prueba?

PATIENT: How are you going to do the test?

MÉDICO: Vamos a inyectar una tinta por un catéter que es un tubo que vamos a insertar en el conducto biliar. Después, vamos a hacer las radiografías.

DOCTOR: We are going to insert a dye through a catheter, which is a tube that we are going to insert in your bile duct. Afterwards we are going to take the X-rays.

PACIENTE: ¿Me va a doler mucho? ¿Habrá efectos secundarios?

PATIENT: Will it hurt much? Will there be side effects?

MÉDICO: El tubo le va a molestar un poco. Posiblemente se sentirá débil y tendrá náuseas después del procedimiento.

DOCTOR: The tube will bother you a little bit. Possibly you will be weak and feel nauseous after the procedure.

PACIENTE: ¿Hay algún riesgo?

PATIENT: Is there any risk?

MÉDICO: Siempre habrá la posibilidad de infección, fiebre, y aún hemorragia.

DOCTOR: There is always the possibility of infection, fever, and even bleeding.

QUESTIONS ON CONVERSATION

1. ¿Por qué van a hacer las radiografías de la vesícula biliar del paciente?
2. ¿Qué quieren determinar los médicos?
3. ¿Cómo van a hacer el procedimiento?

4. ¿Le va a doler al paciente el catéter?
5. ¿Habrá efectos secundarios?
6. ¿Habrá cierto riesgo?

Written practice

Translate the sentences into Spanish.

1. The doctors think that I have gallstones.
2. They will have to operate soon.
3. He says that I'm going to be nauseous after the tests.
4. They will need to examine the results of the X-rays.
5. Will I be very weak?

Vocabulary

NUCLEAR SCANNING: LIVER AND GALLBLADDER
LA EXPLORACIÓN NUCLEAR: EL HÍGADO Y LA VESÍCULA BILIAR

las anormalidades *abnormalities*
las fotos *photos*
la materia radioactiva *radioactive material*

quedarse acostado *to remain lying down*
registrar la señal *to pick up the signal*

Conversation

PACIENTE: ¿Qué me va a hacer?

DOCTORA: Vamos a inyectar materia radioactiva en el brazo. Después de hacer esto, vamos a usar una máquina que producirá fotos del hígado y de la vesícula biliar. De esta manera podremos examinar estos órganos para determinar si hay anormalidades.

PACIENTE: ¿Me va a doler?

DOCTORA: No, pero tiene que quedarse acostado por muchas horas. La máquina no le hará nada a Ud. Sólo registrará la señal de la materia radioactiva.

PATIENT: What are you going to do to me?

DOCTOR: We are going to inject a radioactive material in your arm. After doing this we are going to use a machine that will make photos of your liver and gallbladder. In this way we will be able to examine these organs in order to determine if there are any abnormalities.

PATIENT: Is it going to hurt?

DOCTOR: No, but you have to remain lying down for many hours. The machine will not do anything to you. It just picks up the signal from the radioactive material.

QUESTIONS ON CONVERSATION

1. ¿Qué van a insertar en el brazo del paciente?
2. ¿Qué producirá la máquina?
3. ¿Qué piensan determinar los médicos?
4. ¿Cuál es la función de la máquina?
5. ¿Le va a doler al paciente este procedimiento?

Written practice

Translate the sentences into Spanish.

1. They are going to inject radioactive material into my arm.
2. They have found abnormalities in my liver.
3. They examined my gallbladder.
4. The machine picked up the signal.
5. They used a special machine that makes pictures.

Vocabulary

NUCLEAR SCANNING: PANCREAS
LA EXPLORACION NUCLEAR: EL PÁNCREAS

la cámara *camera*
el quiste *cyst*
una reacción alérgica *an allergic reaction*

sacar fotos *to take photos*
la substancia radioactiva *radioactive substance*

Conversation

MÉDICO: Vamos a tratar de determinar si Ud. tiene quistes en el páncreas.

DOCTOR: We are going to try to determine if you have cysts in your pancreas.

PACIENTE: ¿Qué piensan hacer Uds.?

PATIENT: What do you intend to do?

MÉDICO: Vamos a ponerle una inyección de substancia radioactiva en el brazo. Después, vamos a sacar fotos del órgano con una cámara especial.

DOCTOR: We are going to inject a radioactive substance into your arm. Later, we are going to take photographs of the organ with a special camera.

PACIENTE: ¿Me va a doler?

PATIENT: Is it going to hurt?

MÉDICO: No le va a doler. Posiblemente, después del procedimiento, tendrá una reacción alérgica a la substancia radioactiva.

DOCTOR: It is not going to hurt you. Possibly, after the procedure, you will have an allergic reaction to the radioactive substance.

QUESTIONS ON CONVERSATION

1. ¿Qué piensa determinar el médico?
2. ¿Qué tipo de substancia van a inyectar en el brazo del paciente?
3. ¿Le va a doler al paciente?
4. ¿De qué órgano van a sacar las fotos?
5. ¿Qué tipo de reacción va a sufrir el paciente?

Written practice

Translate the sentences into Spanish.

1. I have cysts in my pancreas.
2. Why did they inject radioactive material into my arm?
3. Is this a dangerous procedure?
4. He had an allergic reaction.
5. This special camera took pictures of my pancreas.

Vocabulary

ULTRASOUND MACHINE/LA MÁQUINA ULTRASONIDO

el aparato *device, machine*
penetrar *to penetrate*
producido,-a por *produced by*

el transmisor ultrasonido *ultrasound transmitter*
transmitir *to transmit*

Conversation

DOCTORA: Tenemos que examinarle el hígado.

DOCTOR: We have to examine your liver.

PACIENTE: ¿Por qué? ¿Cuál es el problema?

PATIENT: Why? What is the problem?

DOCTORA: Queremos determinar si hay tumores en este órgano.

DOCTOR: We want to determine if there are tumors in this organ.

PACIENTE: ¿Qué es este aparato que me está poniendo sobre el estómago? Tengo miedo.

PATIENT: What is this device that you are putting on my stomach? I'm afraid.

DOCTORA: Cálmese señor. El aparato que estoy usando no le penetrará la piel. Sólo va a transmitir sonidos producidos por el hígado. Se llama un transmisor ultrasonido. De esta manera, podemos estudiar este órgano y hacer un diagnóstico.

DOCTOR: Calm down, sir. The device that I am using will not penetrate the skin. It is just going to transmit sounds produced by your liver. It is called an ultrasound transmitter. In this way we can study the organ and make a diagnosis.

QUESTIONS ON CONVERSATION

1. ¿Qué órgano van a examinar?
2. ¿Qué quieren determinar?
3. ¿De qué tiene miedo el paciente?
4. ¿Qué transmitirá el aparato?
5. ¿Cómo se llama el aparato?

Written practice

Translate the sentences into Spanish.

1. He is afraid of all these devices.
2. It is necessary to determine what the problem is.
3. We have found tumors in his liver.
4. The doctors examined his liver.
5. He used an ultrasound transmitter.

Vocabulary

URINE COLLECTION/EL DEPÓSITO DE LA ORINA

correr el riesgo   *to run the risk*
incómodo,-a *uncomfortable*
irritar *to irritate*

sacar la orina   *to remove urine*
la sonda   *catheter*

Conversation

MÉDICO: Tenemos que insertar una sonda por la uretra hasta la vejiga para sacar la orina.

DOCTOR: We have to insert a catheter through your urethra up to the bladder in order to remove urine.

PACIENTE: ¿Me va a doler?

PATIENT: Is it going to hurt?

MÉDICO: Se sentirá incómoda porque la sonda le va a irritar.

DOCTOR: You will feel uncomfortable because the catheter is going to irritate you.

PACIENTE: ¿Hay la posibilidad de complicaciones?

PATIENT: Is there the possibility of complications?

MÉDICO: Sí, corremos el riesgo de infección. Pero no se preocupe, no es nada grave.

DOCTOR: Yes, we run the risk of infection. But don't worry, it's nothing serious.

QUESTIONS ON CONVERSATION

1. ¿Por qué van a insertar el catéter en la vejiga de la paciente?
2. ¿Cómo se sentirá la paciente?

3. ¿Qué le va a irritar a la paciente?
4. ¿Habrá complicaciones?
5. ¿Es grave la situación?

Written practice

Translate the sentences into Spanish.

1. They are going to remove the urine from the bladder.
2. The catheter is going to bother you.
3. I know that I'm running the risk of infection.
4. Will I feel a lot of pain?
5. How can we avoid complications?

Vocabulary

INTRAVENOUS PYELOGRAM/EL PIELOGRAMA INTRAVENOSO

a lo mejor *perhaps*
las piedras nefríticas *kidney stones*
proponerse a *to propose to*

la tinta *dye*
el yodo *iodine*

Conversation

MÉDICO: Le vamos a inyectar una tinta de yodo en el brazo. Después, vamos a hacer unas radiografías de los riñones. El procedimiento se llama un pielograma intravenoso.

DOCTOR: We are going to inject an iodine dye into your arm. Later on, we are going to take some X-rays of your kidneys. The procedure is called an intravenous pyelogram.

PACIENTE: ¿Qué se propone a determinar con esta prueba?

PATIENT: What do you propose to determine with this test?

MÉDICO: Queremos determinar si hay quistes o piedras nefríticas.

DOCTOR: We want to determine if there are cysts or kidney stones.

PACIENTE: ¿Es grave la situación?

PATIENT: Is the situation serious?

MÉDICO: No se preocupe Ud. A lo mejor sólo tiene una infección de los riñones.

DOCTOR: Don't worry. Perhaps you only have a kidney infection.

QUESTIONS ON CONVERSATION

1. ¿Qué van a inyectar en el brazo del paciente?
2. ¿De qué órgano van a hacer las radiografías?
3. ¿Qué piensan determinar con estas pruebas?
4. ¿Qué le pregunta el paciente al médico?
5. ¿Por qué no debe preocuparse el paciente?

Written practice

Translate the sentences into Spanish.

1. They injected an iodine dye into my arm.
2. They found out that I have kidney stones.
3. He is suffering from a kidney infection.
4. They took X-rays of my kidneys.
5. He is trying to cure the patient.

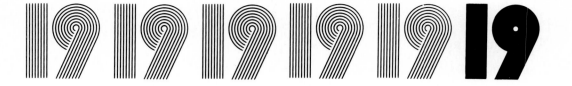

Vocabulary

THE DENTIST/EL DENTISTA

absceso   *abscess*
adormecer el nervio   *to deaden the nerve*
el anestético local   *local anesthetic*
el bicúspide   *bicuspid*
la carie   *cavity*
cepillarse los dientes   *to brush one's teeth*
el cepillo de dientes   *toothbrush*
el cielo de la boca   *roof of the mouth*
la clínica dental   *dental clinic*
el colmillo   *eyetooth*
la corona   *crown*
cubrir   *to cover*
de abajo   *lower*
de arriba   *upper*
la dentadura postiza   *denture*
la dentadura completa   *full denture*
la dentadura parcial   *partial denture*
el diente cariado   *a decayed tooth*
los dientes de leche   *baby teeth*
el dolor de dientes   *toothache*
el dolor de muelas   *toothache*
empastar   *to fill*
el empaste   *filling*
las encías inflamadas   *inflamed gums*

enjuagarse   *to rinse*
escupir en la taza   *to spit in the cup*
el esmalte   *enamel*
la extracción   *extraction*
extraer   *to extract*
el gas   *gas*
los incisivos   *incisors*
la infección de las encías   *gum infection*
la lengua   *tongue*
limpiar los dientes   *to clean the teeth*
la limpieza   *cleaning*
masticar   *to chew*
la muela del juicio impactado   *impacted wisdom tooth*
obstruir el nervio   *to obstruct the nerve*
el paladar   *palate*
la piorrea   *pyhorrea*
el puente   *bridge*
la raíz   *root*
la saliva   *saliva*
sangrarle (a uno)   *to bleed*
taladrar   *to drill*
el taladro   *drill*
los tratamientos   *treatments*

Oral practice

Change the sentences using the cues.

1. El dentista tiene que extraer el diente.
   - deaden the nerve   • clean my teeth   • use a local anesthetic   • drill the tooth
   - give me several treatments

2. El paciente tiene que cepillarse los dientes.
   - rinse his mouth   • spit in the cup   • sit in the chair   • open his mouth
   - close his mouth

3. El dentista va a extraer el diente.
   - a bicuspid   • a decayed tooth   • a baby tooth   • a wisdom tooth
   - an incisor

4. Tendré que visitar al dentista porque me duele un diente.
   - I have a decayed tooth   • I need a partial denture   • I need a filling
   - I have inflamed gums   • I need a gum treatment

Answer the questions with complete sentences.

1. ¿Visita Ud. al dentista regularmente?
2. ¿Se cepilla Ud. los dientes después de cada comida?
3. ¿Le molesta a Ud. la dentadura postiza?
4. ¿Tiene Ud. las encías inflamadas?
5. ¿Necesita Ud. un cepillo de dientes?
6. ¿Cuánto tiempo hace que tiene Ud. dolor de diente?
7. ¿Toma Ud. algo para la infección de las encías?
8. ¿Se enjuaga Ud. la boca con agua?
9. ¿Le sangran mucho las encías?
10. ¿Cuántas visitas tiene Ud. que hacer a la clínica dental?

Answer the questions with complete sentences.

1. ¿Ha adormecido el nervio el dentista?
2. ¿Ha obstruido el nervio la dentista?
3. ¿Ha extraído el bicúspide el dentista?
4. ¿Ha taladrado el diente la dentista?
5. ¿Ha usado un anestético local el dentista?
6. ¿Ha empastado la carie el dentista?
7. ¿Ha tratado la infección el dentista?
8. ¿Ha consultado la dentista con los padres del niño?
9. ¿Ha sacado las radiografías el dentista?
10. ¿Le ha dado la receta el dentista?

Written practice

Translate the sentences into Spanish.

1. I must extract an impacted wisdom tooth.
2. The dentist is going to do three fillings today.
3. This extraction will hurt very much without a local anesthetic.
4. The dentist says that I need a partial denture.
5. You should visit the dental clinic.
6. You have many cavities because you do not brush your teeth.
7. I must drill the cavity before filling it.
8. Rinse and spit in the cup, please.
9. You have pain in your mouth because your gums are inflamed.
10. Open your mouth, please.

Conversations

A: Me duele mucho un diente.

B: Indique donde le duele.

A: Aquí en la parte de atrás es donde duele.

B: Esa es una muela del juicio. Está impactada y tengo que extraerla.

A: ¿Me va a poner un anestético?

B: Sí, le voy a poner una inyección de pentotal.

A: ¿Cuánto tiempo hace que Ud. no visita al dentista?

B: Hace dos años.

A: Eso es mucho tiempo.

B: He estado muy ocupado. ¿Cuántas caries tengo?

A: Ud. tiene seis caries.

B: Favor de empastar dos ahora, y volveré en una semana.

A: One of my teeth hurts a lot.

B: Show me where it hurts.

A: Here in the back is where it hurts.

B: That is a wisdom tooth. It is impacted and I must extract it.

A: Are you going to give me an anesthetic?

B: Yes, I am going to give you an injection of pentothal.

A: How long has it been since you last visited the dentist?

B: It has been two years.

A: That is a long time.

B: I have been very busy. How many cavities do I have?

A: You have six cavities.

B: Please fill two now, and I will come back in a week.

Vocabulary

GYNECOLOGY/LA GINECOLOGÍA

el aborto espontáneo *accidental abortion*

el aborto provocado *planned abortion*

el cáncer *cancer*

el coito *coitus*

el condón *condom*

los contraceptivos   *contraceptives*
el diafragma   *diaphragm*
la dificultad al orinar   *difficulty urinating*
las drogas   *drugs*
las duchas   *douches*
durar   *to last*
el embarazo   *pregnancy*
las enfermedades venéreas   *venereal diseases*
el flujo   *discharge*
el ginecólogo, la ginecóloga   *gynecologist*
la gonorrea   *gonorrhea*

la hemorragia   *hemorrhage*
la histerectomía   *hysterectomy*
menstruar   *to menstruate*
la operación cesárea   *caesarian operation*
la pelvis estrecha   *narrow pelvis*
el período, la regla   *menstrual period*
el período regular, irregular   *regular, irregular period*
la píldora   *the pill*
las relaciones sexuales   *sexual relations*
sangrar   *to bleed*
la sífilis   *syphilis*

Oral practice

Change the sentences using the cues.

1. La paciente ha tenido un aborto espontáneo.
   - a planned abortion   • difficulty urinating   • a hysterectomy
   - irregular periods   • a hemorrhage

2. La paciente ha usado contraceptivos.
   - a diaphragm   • douches   • the pill   • drugs   • an IUD

3. El ginecólogo dice que la paciente tiene una enfermedad venérea.
   - syphilis   • gonorrhea   • cancer of the cervix   • a narrow pelvis
   - cysts in her ovaries

Answer the questions with complete sentences.

1. ¿Usa Ud. contraceptivos?
2. ¿Necesita Ud. una histerectomía?
3. ¿Tiene Ud. los períodos regulares?
4. ¿Toma Ud. drogas?
5. ¿Consulta Ud. con el ginecólogo?
6. ¿Cuántos días dura su período menstrual?
7. ¿Es su primer embarazo?
8. ¿Sufre Ud. de cáncer?
9. ¿Cuánto tiempo hace que Ud. usa la píldora?
10. ¿Es Ud. casada o soltera?

Answer the questions with complete sentences.

1. ¿Le ha examinado a Ud. el ginecólogo?
2. ¿Le ha recomendado la píldora la ginecóloga?
3. ¿Le ha dicho a Ud. el ginecólogo que tiene sífilis?

4. ¿Le ha recetado algo la ginecóloga para la infección?
5. ¿Le ha dado el diafragma el ginecólogo?
6. ¿Le ha preguntado sobre su historia médica la ginecóloga?
7. ¿Le ha dicho a Ud. el ginecólogo cuál es su problema?
8. ¿Le ha recomendado una histerectomía el ginecólogo?
9. ¿Le ha dicho a Ud. el ginecólogo que está embarazada?
10. ¿Le ha dicho a Ud. la ginecóloga que tiene una enfermedad venérea?

Written practice

Translate the sentences into Spanish.

1. The gynecologist says that I am pregnant.
2. How long have you had difficulty urinating?
3. Your problem is that you have a very narrow pelvis.
4. You should not use the pill.
5. My period has been very irregular.
6. The gynecologist has recommended the use of the diaphragm.
7. The gynecologist says that I have gonorrhea.
8. I am going to have an abortion.
9. You should not take any drugs during your pregnancy.
10. She has been bleeding excessively during her menstrual periods.

Conversations

A: ¿Cuál es su problema?
B: Me duele cada vez que tengo relaciones sexuales.
A: ¿Cuánto tiempo hace que tiene Ud. este problema?
B: Hace unos meses.
A: ¿Sangra Ud. después de tener relaciones sexuales?
B: A veces, sí. ¿Qué puedo hacer, doctor?
A: Voy a hacerle un examen físico para determinar cuál es su problema.

A: What is your problem?
B: It hurts every time I have sexual relations.
A: How long have you had this problem?
B: For a few months.
A: Do you bleed after having sexual relations?
B: Sometimes, yes. What can I do, doctor?
A: I am going to give you a physical exam to determine what your problem is.

A: Doctor, creo que tengo una enfermedad venérea.
B: ¿Por qué dice Ud. esto?
A: Porque tengo flujo de la vagina.

A: Doctor, I think I have a venereal disease.
B: Why do you say this?
A: Because I have a discharge from my vagina.

B: ¿Cuánto tiempo hace que tiene el
flujo?
A: Hace unas semanas.
B: Tendré que examinarle la vagina.

B: How long have you had the
discharge?
A: For a few weeks.
B: I will have to examine your vagina.

Vocabulary

THE OPTOMETRIST / EL OPTOMETRISTA

los anteojos   *eyeglasses*
las armaduras   *frames*
arreglar   *to adjust*
el astigmatismo   *astigmatism*
los bifocales   *bifocals*
borroso,-a   *blurred*
la carta   *chart*
la catarata   *cataract*
claro   *clear*
el daltonismo   *colorblindness*
los espejuelos   *eyeglasses*
examinar   *to examine*
las gafas   *eyeglasses*
las gafas de sol   *sunglasses*
el glaucoma   *glaucoma*
la hipermetropía   *farsightedness*

leer   *to read*
los lentes   *lenses, eyeglasses*
los lentes de contacto   *contact lenses*
la línea   *line*
la luz   *light*
la miopia   *myopia, nearsightedness*
mirar   *to look at*
los ojos   *eyes*
ponerse borroso   *to become blurred*
el puente   *bridge*
la retina   *retina*
tener buena vista   *to have good vision*
usar   *to wear*
ver   *to see*
la vista   *sight*

Oral practice

Change the sentences using the cues.

1. El paciente quiere bifocales.
   • eyeglasses   • new frames   • contact lenses   • new lenses   • sunglasses

2. La paciente debe mirar la carta.
   • read the chart   • read the second line   • visit the optometrist
   • wear the glasses   • clean his glasses

3. El optometrista va a preparar los bifocales.
   • examine my eyes   • prepare the prescription   • adjust the frames
   • recommend contact lenses   • change the lenses

Answer the questions with complete sentences.

1. ¿Le gustan estas armaduras?
2. ¿Quiere Ud. lentes de contacto?
3. ¿Usa las gafas de sol todo el tiempo?

4. ¿Puede Ud. leer la primera línea de la carta?
5. ¿Tiene buena vista?
6. ¿Le molesta el puente?
7. ¿Tiene Ud. una cita con el optometrista?
8. ¿Tiene Ud. la vista borrosa?
9. ¿Usa Ud. los espejuelos para leer?
10. ¿Quiere Ud. usar los bifocales?

Answer the questions with complete sentences.

1. ¿Le ha examinado los ojos el optometrista?
2. ¿Le ha recomendado los lentes de contacto el optometrista?
3. ¿Le ha arreglado las armaduras el optometrista?
4. ¿Ha preparado las gafas el optometrista?
5. ¿Le ha dado las gafas de sol el optometrista?
6. ¿Le ha dicho el optometrista cuál es su problema?
7. ¿Ha encontrado los lentes correctos el optometrista?
8. ¿Le ha preparado los bifocales el optometrista?
9. ¿Le ha dado a Ud. el optometrista las armaduras que prefiere?
10. ¿Le ha preparado la receta el optometrista?

Written practice

Translate the sentences into Spanish.

1. The optometrist is examining my eyes.
2. I want to wear contact lenses.
3. I do not like these frames.
4. Please read the second line on the chart.
5. You have very good vision, Mr. García.
6. I am going to make an appointment with the optometrist.
7. I need a new prescription.
8. You should not wear sunglasses all the time.
9. My vision is becoming very blurred.
10. I have to adjust the bridge on these glasses.

Conversations

A: ¿Va a examinarme Ud. los ojos ahora?

B: Sí, pase, por favor. Mire esta carta y dígame lo que ve.

A: ¿Tengo buena vista?

B: No, Ud. no tiene buena vista. Necesita espejuelos.

A: ¿Cuándo estarán listos los espejuelos?

B: Estarán listos en unas horas.

A: Are you going to examine my eyes now?

B: Yes, come in, please. Look at this chart and tell me what you see.

A: Do I have good vision?

B: No, you do not have good vision. You need glasses.

A: When will the glasses be ready?

B: They will be ready in a few hours.

A: Lea la segunda línea, por favor.
B: O, F, D, P, R.
A: Lea la tercera línea.
B: E, C, U, B, Z, F, G.
A: Ahora lea la cuarta línea.
B: La cuarta línea está borrosa.
A: ¿No puede ver ninguna letra en la cuarta línea?
B: No, todo se pone borroso después de la tercera línea.

A: Read the second line, please.
B: O, F, D, P, R.
A: Read the third line.
B: E, C, U, B, Z, F, G.
A: Now read the fourth line.
B: The fourth line is blurred.
A: You can't see any letter on the fourth line?
B: No, everything becomes blurred after the third line.

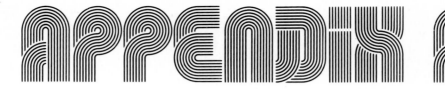

Everyday greetings and expressions of courtesy

Spanish	English
¡Hola!	Hello!
Buenos días.	Good morning.
Buenas tardes.	Good afternoon.
Buenas noches.	Good night.
Perdón; Perdóneme Ud.	Pardon; Pardon me.
Con su permiso.	Excuse me.
Pase Ud. — *Adelante.* — *Entre*	Come in.
Permítame presentarme. *Soy _____*	Allow me to introduce myself.
Encantado,-a. *Me llamo _____*	Pleased (to meet you).
Mucho gusto.	It's a pleasure.
Siéntese, por favor.	Sit down, please.
¿Habla Ud. inglés?	Do you speak English?
¿Me comprende Ud.? *¿entiende (more commonly used)*	Do you understand me?
¿Cuál es su problema? *(tú) -chica*	What is your problem?
¿En qué puedo servirle? *¿ayudarle (te)*	How can I help you?
Lo siento mucho.	I'm very sorry.
¿Cómo está Ud. hoy?	How are you today?
¿Cómo se siente Ud. hoy?	How do you feel today?
¿Cómo le va?	How are you doing?
¿Qué le pasa a Ud.?	What's happening to you?
★ ¿Qué tal?	How are you?
¿Qué tal su familia?	How is your family?
Bien, gracias, ¿y Ud.?	Fine, thanks, and you?
Hasta luego.	See you later.
Hasta mañana.	See you tomorrow.
Hasta la vista.	See you later.
Hasta la próxima cita.	Until the next appointment.

208

★ Qué tal in front of a noun means "how's"
mejor - better
peor - worse

Adiós.   Goodbye.
Gracias.   Thank you.
De nada; No hay de qué.   You're welcome.

Admissions and general information

¿Cómo se llama Ud.? *-su nombre*   What is your name?
¿Cuál es su dirección? *-domecitto -direction*   What is your address?
¿Dónde vive Ud.?   Where do you live?
¿Cuál es la zona postal?   What is the zip code?
¿Cuál es su número de teléfono?   What is your telephone number?
¿Dónde nació Ud.?   Where were you born?
¿Es Ud. ciudadano *(a)* americano?   Are you an American citizen?
¿Cuándo nació Ud.? *fecha de nacimiento? / Where were you born?*   When were you born?
¿Qué edad tiene Ud.?   What is your age?
¿Cuántos años tiene Ud.?   How old are you?
¿Es Ud. soltero,-a?   Are you single?
¿Es Ud. casado,-a?   Are you married?
¿Es Ud. divorciado,-a?   Are you divorced?
¿Es Ud. separado,-a?   Are you separated?
¿Es Ud. viudo?   Are you a widower?
¿Es Ud. viuda?   Are you a widow?
¿Cuál es su religión?   What is your religion?
¿Tiene Ud. trabajo?   Do you have a job?
¿Cuál es su trabajo?   What is your job?
¿Qué trabajo hace Ud.?   What work do you do?
¿En qué trabaja Ud.?   What work do you do?
¿Quién es su pariente (familiar) más   Who is your nearest relative?
   cercano?
¿Tiene Ud. seguro? *(laseguranza)*   Do you have insurance?
¿Cuál es su compañía de seguro?   What is your insurance company?
¿Tiene Ud. Medicare?   Do you have Medicare?
¿Tiene Ud. Medicaid?   Do you have Medicaid?
¿Tiene Ud. un médico de familia?   Do you have a family doctor?
¿Están vivos sus padres?   Are your parents living?
¿Están muertos sus padres?   Are your parents deceased?
¿Cómo murió su madre?   How did your mother die?
¿Cómo murió su padre?   How did your father die?
¿Tiene Ud. hermanos?   Do you have any brothers or sisters?
¿Cuántos años tiene su esposo (esposa)? How old is your husband (wife)? *esposas -handcuffs*
¿Tiene Ud. hijos? *marido / mujer*   Do you have any children?
¿Cuántos años tienen sus hijos?   How old are your children?
¿Ha asistido Ud. a la escuela elemental, Have you attended elementary school,
   secundaria, a la universidad?   high school, college?

¿Cuál es su nombre apellido?   What is your last name?

Commands

Abra la boca.	Open your mouth.
Vaya (Acérquese) a la máquina.	Go up to the machine.
Acuéstese boca abajo (arriba).	Lie face down (up).
Agárrese de la barra.	Hold on to the bar.
Aplíquese esto.	Apply this.
Beba esto.	Drink this.
Cálmese. *Tranquílese.*	Calm down.
Cambie el vendaje.	Change the dressing.
Camine despacio.	Walk slowly.
Coma ahora.	Eat now.
Consulte con el especialista.	Consult with the specialist.
Stop (Deje de) fumar.	Stop smoking.
Déjeme registrarle el pulso (tomarle la temperatura, la presión).	Let me take your pulse (take your temperature, your pressure).
Desnúdese (Desvístase), por favor.	Please undress.
Diga, ''Ah''.	Say, ''Ah''.
Dígame . . .	Tell me . . .
Dóblese hacia adelante (hacia atrás).	Bend forward (backward).
Doble la cabeza a la derecha (a la izquierda).	Bend your head to the right (to the left).
Duerma más.	Sleep more.
Enséñeme dónde le duele.	Show me where it hurts.
Escriba su dirección.	Write your address.
Espere aquí (en la sala de espera, etc.).	Wait here (in the waiting room, etc.).
Firme la autorización (para la cirugía).	Sign the authorization (for the surgery).
Haga un puño.	Make a fist.
Indíqueme dónde le duele.	Show me where it hurts.
Llámeme por teléfono.	Phone me.
Llene los formularios (las recetas).	Fill out the forms (Fill the prescriptions).
Levántese.	Get up.
Levante los brazos (las piernas, etc.).	Raise your arms (legs, etc.).
Mantenga la respiración.	Hold your breath.
Mastique las píldoras.	Chew the pills.
Mire hacia arriba (abajo).	Look up (down).
Muéstreme dónde le duele.	Show me where it hurts.
Mueva los pies (los dedos de los pies).	Move your feet (toes, etc.).
No se mueva.	Don't move.
No se preocupe.	Don't worry.
No se queje tanto.	Don't complain so much.
No tenga miedo.	Don't be afraid.
Pague ahora (en la oficina, etc.).	Pay now (in the office, etc.).
Párese (Póngase de pie).	Stand up.
Put yourself (Póngase) la ropa (la blusa, la camisa, etc.).	Put on your clothes (blouse, shirt, etc.).

No se mueva. — Don't move

Quítate (chila)

Quítese la ropa.   Take off your clothes.
Respire profund~~amente~~.   Breathe deeply.
Salga temprano.   Leave early.
Saque la lengua. *y dice "ahhh"*   Stick out your tongue. *(y say ahhh)*
Señáleme dónde le duele.   Show me where it hurts.
Siéntese. *Tome asciento.*   Sit down.
Siga la dieta (las instrucciones). *báscula*   Follow the diet (the instructions).
Súbase a la mesa (en la ~~balanza~~).   Get on the table (the scale).
Tenga cuidado. *Bájese de la mesa -*   Be careful.
           Get down from the table
Tome esta medicina.   Take this medicine.
Toque el timbre.   Ring the bell.
Tosa.   Cough.
Trague esto.   Swallow this.
Trate de mover las piernas (los brazos,   Try to move your legs (arms, etc.).
   etc.).
Vaya a la clínica, (a la farmacia, etc.).   Go to the clinic, (to the pharmacy, etc.).
Venga mañana (pasado mañana, etc.).   Come tomorrow (the day after tomorrow,
Regrese   etc.).
~~Vuelva~~ en una semana (en un mes, etc.).   Return in a week (in a month, etc.).
~~Vuélvase~~ a la derecha (a la izquierda).   Turn to the right (left).
   ~~Rega~~ *Doble (when walking and driving)*

General questions about health: present illness, past illness, accidents, diseases

¿Tiene dolor?   Are you in pain?
¿Dónde tiene dolor?   Where do you have pain?
¿Qué le duele?   What is hurting you?
¿Qué le pasó?   What happened to you?
¿Tuvo un accidente?   Did you have an accident?
¿Se desmayó?   Did you faint?
¿Perdió el conocimiento?   Did you lose consciousness?
¿Se cayó?   Did you fall?
¿Cómo se cayó?   How did you fall?
¿Dónde se cayó?   Where did you fall?
¿Está bajo tratamiento de un médico?   Are you under doctor's care?
¿Duerme bien?   Do you sleep well?
¿Fuma mucho?   Do you smoke a lot?
¿Está tomando medicinas?   Are you taking medicine?
¿Toma bebidas alcohólicas?   Do you drink alcoholic beverages?
¿Toma drogas?   Are you on drugs?
¿Se cansa fácilmente?   Do you tire easily?
¿Tiene calor?   Are you warm?
¿Tiene catarro?   Do you have a cold?
¿Tiene fiebre (calentura)?   Do you have a fever?

¿Tiene frío? — Are you cold?

¿Tiene hambre? — Are you hungry?

¿Tiene hinchazón en las piernas (en los tobillos, etc.)? — Do you have swelling in your legs (ankles, etc.)? (Are your legs swollen?)

¿Tiene irritación de la piel? — Do you have skin irritation?

¿Tiene mareos? — Are you dizzy?

¿Tiene náusea? — Are you nauseous?

¿Tiene nerviosidad? — Are you nervous?

¿Tiene sangre en la expectoración (en la orina)? — Do you have blood in your expectoration (in your urine)?

¿Tiene sed? — Are you thirsty?

¿Tiene tos? — Do you have a cough?

¿Tiene tos con flema? — Do you have a cough with phlegm?

¿Tiene diarrea? — Do you have diarrhea?

¿Está estreñido,-a? — Are you constipated?

¿Tiene problemas con la digestión (la respiración)? — Do you have digestive (respiratory) problems?

¿Sufre de enfermedades del corazón (de los pulmones, de los riñones)? — Do you suffer from heart (lung, kidney) disease?

¿Sufre de enfermedades venéreas? — Do you suffer from venereal diseases?

¿Sufre de catarros frecuentes? — Do you suffer from frequent colds?

¿Sufre de bronquitis? — Do you suffer from bronchitis?

¿Sufre de laringitis? — Do you suffer from laryngitis?

¿Sufre de cáncer? — Are you suffering from cancer?

¿Sufre de leucemia? — Are you suffering from leukemia?

¿Sufre de los nervios? — Are you suffering from nervousness?

¿Sufre de la presión alta (baja)? — Are you suffering from high blood pressure (low blood pressure)?

¿Sufre de úlceras? — Are you suffering from ulcers?

¿Sufrió un ataque al corazón? — Did you have a heart attack?

¿Ha tenido (padecido de, sufrido de) alergias? — Have you had (suffered from) allergies?

    anemia? — anemia?

    apendicitis? — appendicitis?

    artritis? — arthritis?

    asma? — asthma?

    bursitis? — bursitis?

    cólera? — cholera?

    colitis? — colitis?

    diabetis? — diabetes?

    difteria? — diphtheria?

    disentería? — dysentery?

    epilepsia? — epilepsy?

    fiebre amarilla? — yellow fever?

fiebre de heno?	hay fever?
fiebre reumática?	rheumatic fever?
gonorrea?	gonorrhea?
hepatitis?	hepatitis?
ictericia?	jaundice?
malaria?	malaria?
meningitis?	meningitis?
paperas?	mumps?
pleuresía?	pleurisy?
pulmonía?	pneumonia?
rubéola?	rubella, German measles?
sarampión?	measles?
sífilis?	syphilis?
tifoidea?	typhoid fever?
tos ferina?	whooping cough?
tuberculosis?	tuberculosis?
viruela?	smallpox?
viruelas locas (varicela)?	chicken pox?

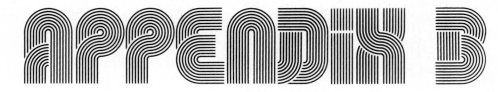

Verbs and Tenses

Present indicative tense

REGULAR -AR VERBS

hablar, *to speak:* **hablo,** *I speak, I am speaking, I do speak*

yo	**hablo**	*I speak*
él/ella	**habla**	*he/she speaks*
Ud.	**habla**	*you speak*
nosotros/nosotras	**hablamos**	*we speak*
ellos/ellas	**hablan**	*they speak*
Uds.	**hablan**	*you (pl.) speak*

REGULAR -ER VERBS

comer, *to eat:* **como,** *I eat, I am eating, I do eat*

yo	**como**	*I eat*
él/ella	**come**	*he/she eats*
Ud.	**come**	*you eat*
nosotros/nosotras	**comemos**	*we eat*
ellos/ellas	**comen**	*they eat*
Uds.	**comen**	*you (pl.) eat*

REGULAR -IR VERBS

vivir, *to live:* **vivo,** *I live, I do live, I am living*

yo	**vivo**	*I live*
él/ella	**vive**	*he/she lives*
Ud.	**vive**	*you live*
nosotros/nosotras	**vivimos**	*we live*
ellos/ellas	**viven**	*they live*
Uds.	**viven**	*you (pl.) live*

VERBS IRREGULAR ONLY IN THE FIRST PERSON SINGULAR

caer	*to fall*	caigo	cae	caemos	caen
conocer	*to know*	conozco	conoce	conocemos	conocen
dar	*to give*	doy	da	damos	dan
hacer	*to do, make*	hago	hace	hacemos	hacen
ofrecer	*to offer*	ofrezco	ofrece	ofrecemos	ofrecen
padecer	*to suffer*	padezco	padece	padecemos	padecen
poner	*to put, place*	pongo	pone	ponemos	ponen
saber	*to know*	sé	sabe	sabemos	saben
salir	*to leave*	salgo	sale	salimos	salen
ver	*to see*	veo	ve	vemos	ven

OTHER IRREGULAR VERBS

acostar	*to put to bed*	acuesto	acuesta	acostamos	acuestan
almorzar	*to have lunch*	almuerzo	almuerza	almorzamos	almuerzan
cerrar	*to close*	cierro	cierra	cerramos	cierran
contar	*to count*	cuento	cuenta	contamos	cuentan
costar	*to cost*	—	cuesta	—	cuestan
decir	*to say, tell*	digo	dice	decimos	dicen
despertar	*to awaken*	despierto	despierta	despertamos	despiertan
doler	*to hurt*	—	duele	—	duelen
dormir	*to sleep*	duermo	duerme	dormimos	duermen
encender	*to light*	enciendo	enciende	encendemos	encienden
entender	*to understand*	entiendo	entiende	entendemos	entienden
estar	*to be*	estoy	está	estamos	están
ir	*to go*	voy	va	vamos	van
morir	*to die*	muero	muere	morimos	mueren

mostrar	*to show*	muestro	muestra	mostramos	muestran
mover	*to move*	muevo	mueve	movemos	mueven
pensar	*to think*	pienso	piensa	pensamos	piensan
perder	*to lose*	pierdo	pierde	perdemos	pierden
poder	*to be able*	puedo	puede	podemos	pueden
preferir	*to prefer*	prefiero	prefiere	preferimos	prefieren
querer	*to wish, want*	quiero	quiere	queremos	quieren
seguir	*to follow*	sigo	sigue	seguimos	siguen
sentir	*to feel*	siento	siente	sentimos	sienten
ser	*to be*	soy	es	somos	son
tener	*to have*	tengo	tiene	tenemos	tienen
venir	*to come*	vengo	viene	venimos	vienen
volver	*to return*	vuelvo	vuelve	volvemos	vuelven

Preterite tense

REGULAR -AR VERBS

hablar, *to speak:* **hablé,** *I spoke*

yo	**hablé**	*I spoke*
él/ella	**habló**	*he/she spoke*
Ud.	**habló**	*you spoke*
nosotros/nosotras	**hablamos**	*we spoke*
ellos/ellas	**hablaron**	*they spoke*
Uds.	**hablaron**	*you* (pl.) *spoke*

REGULAR -ER VERBS

comer, *to eat:* **comí,** *I ate*

yo	**comí**	*I ate*
él/ella	**comió**	*he/she ate*
Ud.	**comió**	*you ate*
nosotros/nosotras	**comimos**	*we ate*
ellos/ellas	**comieron**	*they ate*
Uds.	**comieron**	*you* (pl.) *ate*

REGULAR -IR VERBS

vivir, *to live:* **viví,** *I lived*

yo	**viví**	*I lived*
él/ella	**vivió**	*he/she lived*
Ud.	**vivió**	*you lived*
nosotros/nosotras	**vivimos**	*we lived*
ellos/ellas	**vivieron**	*they lived*
Uds.	**vivieron**	*you* (pl.) *lived*

VERBS IRREGULAR ONLY IN THE FIRST PERSON SINGULAR

aplicar	*to apply*	apliqué	aplicó	aplicamos	aplicaron
buscar	*to look for*	busqué	buscó	buscamos	buscaron
explicar	*to explain*	expliqué	explicó	explicamos	explicaron
indicar	*to indicate*	indiqué	indicó	indicamos	indicaron
llegar	*to arrive*	llegué	llegó	llegamos	llegaron
masticar	*to chew*	mastiqué	masticó	masticamos	masticaron
pagar	*to pay*	pagué	pagó	pagamos	pagaron
sacar	*to take out*	saqué	sacó	sacamos	sacaron
tocar	*to touch*	toqué	tocó	tocamos	tocaron
tragar	*to swallow*	tragué	tragó	tragamos	tragaron

OTHER IRREGULAR VERBS

caer	*to fall*	caí	cayó	caímos	cayeron
creer	*to believe*	creí	creyó	creímos	creyeron
dar	*to give*	di	dio	dimos	dieron
decir	*to say, tell*	dije	dijo	dijimos	dijeron
estar	*to be*	estuve	estuvo	estuvimos	estuvieron
hacer	*to do, make*	hice	hizo	hicimos	hicieron
ir	*to go*	fui	fue	fuimos	fueron
leer	*to read*	leí	leyó	leímos	leyeron
morir	*to die*	morí	murió	morimos	murieron
poder	*to be able*	pude	pudo	pudimos	pudieron
poner	*to put*	puse	puso	pusimos	pusieron
querer	*to wish, want*	quise	quiso	quisimos	quisieron
saber	*to know*	supe	supo	supimos	supieron

seguir	*to follow*	seguí	siguió	seguimos	siguieron
ser	*to be*	fui	fue	fuimos	fueron
tener	*to have*	tuve	tuvo	tuvimos	tuvieron
venir	*to come*	vine	vino	vinimos	vinieron
ver	*to see*	vi	vio	vimos	vieron

Imperfect tense

REGULAR -AR VERBS

hablar, *to speak:* **hablaba,** *I was speaking, I used to speak*

yo	**hablaba**	*I was speaking*
él/ella	**hablaba**	*he/she was speaking*
Ud.	**hablaba**	*you were speaking*
nosotros/nosotras	**hablábamos**	*we were speaking*
ellos/ellas	**hablaban**	*they were speaking*
Uds.	**hablaban**	*you* (pl.) *were speaking*

REGULAR -ER VERBS

comer, *to eat:* **comía,** *I was eating, I used to eat*

yo	**comía**	*I was eating*
él/ella	**comía**	*he/she was eating*
Ud.	**comía**	*you were eating*
nosotros/nosotras	**comíamos**	*we were eating*
ellos/ellas	**comían**	*they were eating*
Uds.	**comían**	*you* (pl.) *were eating*

REGULAR -IR VERBS

vivir, *to live:* **vivía,** *I was living, I used to live*

yo	**vivía**	*I was living*
él/ella	**vivía**	*he/she was living*
Ud.	**vivía**	*you were living*
nosotros/nosotras	**vivíamos**	*we were living*
ellos/ellas	**vivían**	*they were living*
Uds.	**vivían**	*you* (pl.) *were living*

IRREGULAR VERBS

ir	*to go*	iba	iba	íbamos	iban
ser	*to be*	era	era	éramos	eran
ver	*to see*	veía	veía	veíamos	veían

Future tense

REGULAR -AR VERBS

hablar, *to speak:* **hablaré,** *I will speak*

yo	**hablaré**	*I will speak*
él/ella	**hablará**	*he/she will speak*
Ud.	**hablará**	*you will speak*
nosotros/nosotras	**hablaremos**	*we will speak*
ellos/ellas	**hablarán**	*they will speak*
Uds.	**hablarán**	*you (pl.) will speak*

REGULAR -ER VERBS

comer, *to eat:* **comeré,** *I will eat*

yo	**comeré**	*I will eat*
él/ella	**comerá**	*he/she will eat*
Ud.	**comerá**	*you will eat*
nosotros/nosotras	**comeremos**	*we will eat*
ellos/ellas	**comerán**	*they will eat*
Uds.	**comerán**	*you (pl.) will eat*

REGULAR -IR VERBS

vivir, *to live:* **viviré,** *I will live*

yo	**viviré**	*I will live*
él/ella	**vivirá**	*he/she will live*
Ud.	**vivirá**	*you will live*
nosotros/nosotras	**viviremos**	*we will live*
ellos/ellas	**vivirán**	*they will live*
Uds.	**vivirán**	*you (pl.) will live*

IRREGULAR VERBS

decir	*to say, tell*	diré	dirá	diremos	dirán
haber	*to have (aux.)*	habré	habrá	habremos	habrán
hacer	*to do, make*	haré	hará	haremos	harán
poder	*to be able*	podré	podrá	podremos	podrán
poner	*to put, place*	pondré	pondrá	pondremos	pondrán
querer	*to wish, want*	querré	querrá	querremos	querrán
saber	*to know*	sabré	sabrá	sabremos	sabrán

salir	*to leave*	saldré	saldrá	saldremos	saldrán
tener	*to have*	tendré	tendrá	tendremos	tendrán
venir	*to come*	vendré	vendrá	vendremos	vendrán

Present progressive tense

REGULAR -AR VERBS

hablar, *to speak:* **estoy hablando,** *I am speaking*

yo	**estoy hablando**	*I am speaking*
él/ella	**está hablando**	*he/she is speaking*
Ud.	**está hablando**	*you are speaking*
nosotros/nosotras	**estamos hablando**	*we are speaking*
ellos/ellas	**están hablando**	*they are speaking*
Uds.	**están hablando**	*you* (pl.) *are speaking*

REGULAR -ER VERBS

comer, *to eat:* **estoy comiendo,** *I am eating*

yo	**estoy comiendo**	*I am eating*
él/ella	**está comiendo**	*he/she is eating*
Ud.	**está comiendo**	*you are eating*
nosotros/nosotras	**estamos comiendo**	*we are eating*
ellos/ellas	**están comiendo**	*they are eating*
Uds.	**están comiendo**	*you* (pl.) *are eating*

REGULAR -IR VERBS

vivir, *to live:* **estoy viviendo,** *I am living*

yo	**estoy viviendo**	*I am living*
él/ella	**está viviendo**	*he/she is living*
Ud.	**está viviendo**	*you are living*
nosotros/nosotras	**estamos viviendo**	*we are living*
ellos/ellas	**están viviendo**	*they are living*
Uds.	**están viviendo**	*you* (pl.) *are living*

IRREGULAR GERUNDS

caer	*to fall*	**cayendo**	*falling*
creer	*to believe*	**creyendo**	*believing*
decir	*to say, tell*	**diciendo**	*saying, telling*

leer *to read*	**leyendo** *reading*
morir *to die*	**muriendo** *dying*
seguir *to follow*	**siguiendo** *following*
sentir *to feel*	**sintiendo** *feeling*
venir *to come*	**viniendo** *coming*

Present perfect tense

REGULAR -AR VERBS

hablar, *to speak:* **he hablado,** *I have spoken*

yo	**he hablado**	*I have spoken*
él/ella	**ha hablado**	*he/she has spoken*
Ud.	**ha hablado**	*you have spoken*
nosotros/nosotras	**hemos hablado**	*we have spoken*
ellos/ellas	**han hablado**	*they have spoken*
Uds.	**han hablado**	*you* (pl.) *have spoken*

REGULAR -ER VERBS

comer, *to eat:* **he comido,** *I have eaten*

yo	**he comido**	*I have eaten*
él/ella	**ha comido**	*he/she has eaten*
Ud.	**ha comido**	*you have eaten*
nosotros/nosotras	**hemos comido**	*we have eaten*
ellos/ellas	**han comido**	*they have eaten*
Uds.	**han comido**	*you* (pl.) *have eaten*

REGULAR -IR VERBS

vivir, *to live:* **he vivido,** *I have lived*

yo	**he vivido**	*I have lived*
él/ella	**ha vivido**	*he/she has lived*
Ud.	**ha vivido**	*you have lived*
nosotros/nosotras	**hemos vivido**	*we have lived*
ellos/ellas	**han vivido**	*they have lived*
Uds.	**han vivido**	*you* (pl.) *have lived*

IRREGULAR PAST PARTICIPLES

abrir *to open*	**abierto** *opened*
cubrir *to cover*	**cubierto** *covered*

decir *to say, tell*	**dicho** *said, told*
escribir *to write*	**escrito** *written*
hacer *to do, make*	**hecho** *done, made*
morir *to die*	**muerto** *died*
poner *to put, place*	**puesto** *put, placed*
ver *to see*	**visto** *seen*

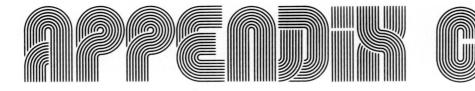

Parts of the Body

THE HEAD / LA CABEZA

(1)   scalp
(2)   hair
(3)   forehead
(4)   eyebrow
(5)   eye
(6)   temple
(7)   (outer) ear
(8)   (inner) ear
(9)   cheek
(10) nose
(11) nostrils
(12) jaw
(13) mouth
(14) chin
(15) neck
(16) Adam's apple

Also:

el cerebro   brain
la nuca   nape of the neck
los párpados   eyelids
las pestañas   eyelashes

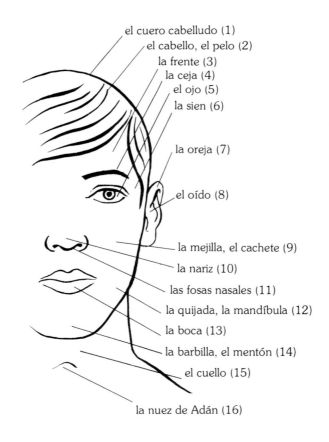

el cuero cabelludo (1)
el cabello, el pelo (2)
la frente (3)
la ceja (4)
el ojo (5)
la sien (6)
la oreja (7)
el oído (8)
la mejilla, el cachete (9)
la nariz (10)
las fosas nasales (11)
la quijada, la mandíbula (12)
la boca (13)
la barbilla, el mentón (14)
el cuello (15)
la nuez de Adán (16)

THE MOUTH / LA BOCA

(1) lip
(2) gums
(3) palate
(4) tonsils
(5) tongue
(6) teeth
(7) wisdom tooth
(8) molar
(9) bicuspid
(10) eyetooth
(11) incisor

Also:

la corona   crown
la dentadura postiva   false teeth
el diente de leche   milk tooth
el puente   bridge

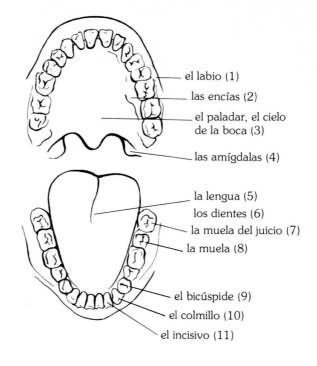

el labio (1)
las encías (2)
el paladar, el cielo de la boca (3)
las amígdalas (4)
la lengua (5)
los dientes (6)
la muela del juicio (7)
la muela (8)
el bicúspide (9)
el colmillo (10)
el incisivo (11)

THE ARM / EL BRAZO

(1) elbow
(2) forearm
(3) wrist
(4) hand
(5) thumb
(6) index finger
(7) middle finger
(8) ring finger
(9) little finger

Also:

el dorso de la mano   the back of the hand
la palma de la mano   palm
el puño   fist
el nudillo   knuckle
la uña   fingernail

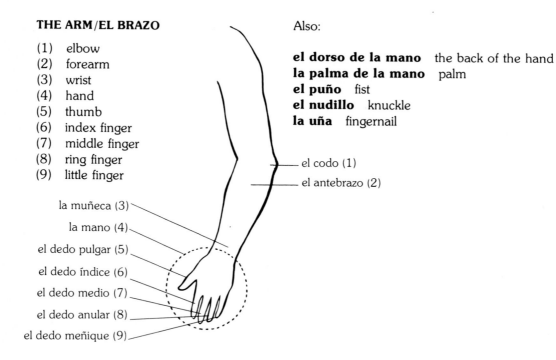

el codo (1)
el antebrazo (2)
la muñeca (3)
la mano (4)
el dedo pulgar (5)
el dedo índice (6)
el dedo medio (7)
el dedo anular (8)
el dedo meñique (9)

THE LEG/LA PIERNA

(1) thigh
(2) kneecap
(3) knee
(4) shin
(5) calf
(6) ankle
(7) foot
(8) heel
(9) sole
(10) instep
(11) toes

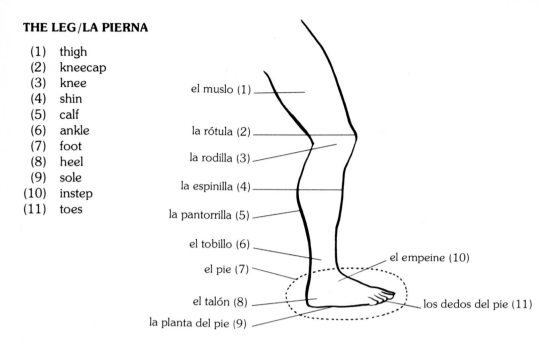

el muslo (1)
la rótula (2)
la rodilla (3)
la espinilla (4)
la pantorrilla (5)
el tobillo (6)
el pie (7)
el talón (8)
la planta del pie (9)
el empeine (10)
los dedos del pie (11)

THE TRUNK/EL TRONCO

(1) shoulder
(2) breast/chest
(3) armpit
(4) nipple
(5) abdomen
(6) waist
(7) navel
(8) crotch
(9) back
(10) hip
(11) buttock

Also:

la barriga belly
el diafragma diaphragm
el tórax thorax
el vientre womb, abdomen

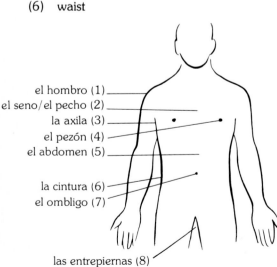

el hombro (1)
el seno/el pecho (2)
la axila (3)
el pezón (4)
el abdomen (5)
la cintura (6)
el ombligo (7)
las entrepiernas (8)
la espalda (9)
la cadera (10)
la nalga (11)

THE DIGESTIVE SYSTEM/EL SISTEMA DIGESTIVO

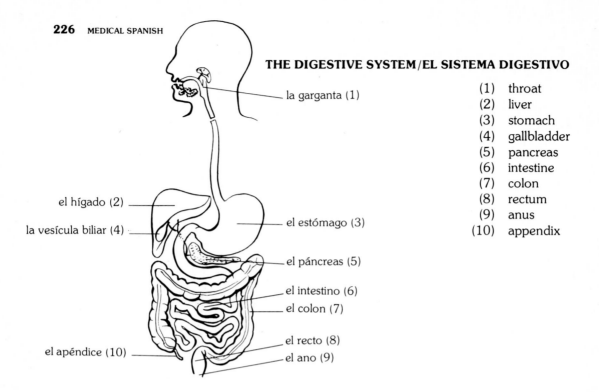

la garganta (1)

el hígado (2)

la vesícula biliar (4)

el estómago (3)

el páncreas (5)

el intestino (6)

el colon (7)

el recto (8)

el ano (9)

el apéndice (10)

(1) throat
(2) liver
(3) stomach
(4) gallbladder
(5) pancreas
(6) intestine
(7) colon
(8) rectum
(9) anus
(10) appendix

THE SKELETON/EL ESQUELETO

(1) skull
(2) collar bone
(3) shoulder blade
(4) rib
(5) breastbone
(6) spinal column
(7) pelvis

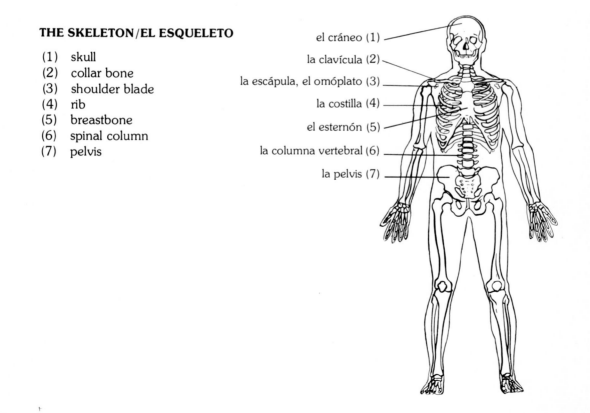

el cráneo (1)

la clavícula (2)

la escápula, el omóplato (3)

la costilla (4)

el esternón (5)

la columna vertebral (6)

la pelvis (7)

OTHER ORGANS/OTROS ÓRGANOS

el bazo, el esplín spleen
los bronquios bronchial tubes
el corazón heart
el cuello uterino, la cerviz cervix
los órganos genitales genital organs
el ovario ovary
el pene, el miembro penis
la piel skin

el pulmón lung
el riñón kidney
la sangre blood
los testículos testicles
el útero, la matriz uterus
la vagina vagina
la vejiga urinary bladder

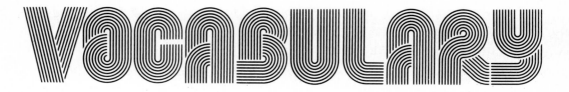

VOCABULARY

These vocabularies are not intended to serve as a dictionary, merely as a guide. They include all of the words identified in the text plus a number of other important medical terms that were not in any of the lessons. The gender of Spanish nouns is indicated only when they do not end in the masculine **-o** or the feminine **-a**. Adjectives ending in **-o** and **-a** are only given in the masculine form.

ABBREVIATIONS

a	adjective	*mf*	common gender
f	feminine	*n*	noun
m	masculine	*pl*	plural

Spanish to English

A

a   at; to

abajo   down; underneath

abandonar   to abandon

abdomen *m*   abdomen

abierto   open

abogado   lawyer

aborto   abortion;
— **accidental** miscarriage; — **provocado** abortion; — **terapéutico** therapeutic abortion

abril *m*   April

abrir   to open

abstenerse   to abstain

abuela   grandmother

abuelo   grandfather; —**s** grandparents

aburrido   bored, boring

acabar   to end, finish; — **de** to have just

accidente *m*   accident

aceite *m*   oil

aceptar   to accept

acercarse (a)   to approach

aconsejar   to advise

acordarse (de)   to remember

acostado   lying down

acostarse   to lie down; go to bed

actitud *f*   attitude

actividad *f*   activity

actor *m*   actor

actriz *f*   actress

adelante   ahead

además   furthermore; — **de** besides, in addition to

adicional   additional

adicto   addict

adiós   goodbye

adoptar   to adopt

adormecer el nervio   to deaden the nerve

adulto   adult

agarrarse (de)   to grab; hold on to

agitado   agitated, excited, nervous

agosto   August

agradable   pleasant

agresivo   aggressive

agrio   bitter

agua   water; — **mineral** mineral water

agudo   sharp

ahogarse   to drown, suffocate

ahora   now; — **mismo** right now

aire *m*   air;
— **acondicionado** air conditioning

al (a + el)   to the

albaricoque *m*   apricot

alcohol *m*   alcohol

alcohólico   alcoholic

alcoholismo   alcoholism

alegre   happy

alergia   allergy

alérgico   allergic

algo   something

alguno   some, any; —**s** some, a few

alimentar   to feed

alimento   food

aliviar   to relieve

almeja   clam

almohada   pillow

almohadilla eléctrica heating pad

almorranas *f pl* hemorrhoids, piles

almorzar   to have lunch

almuerzo   lunch; **tomar el** — to have lunch

alternativa   alternative

alto   tall; high

alucinar   to hallucinate

allí   there

amable   kind, friendly

ama de casa   housewife

ambiente *m*   environment

ambulancia   ambulance

amígdalas *f pl*   tonsils

amigo, -a   friend

amputar   to amputate

analgésico   analgesic

análisis *m*   analysis; **hacer el** — to do the analysis

analizar   to analyze

anatomía   anatomy

anciano, -a *n*   elderly person; *a* elderly, old

anemia anemia
anestesia anesthesia;
— **caudal** caudal
anesthesia; — **general**
general anesthesia; — **local**
local anesthesia
anestesiar to anesthetize
anestesiólogo, -a
anesthesiologist
anestético anesthetic
anfetamina amphetamine
anillo ring
ano anus
anoche last night
anormalidad *f* abnormality
anteayer the day before
yesterday
anteojos *m pl* eyeglasses
antes (de) before
antiácido antacid
antibiótico antibiotic
anticonceptivo
contraceptive
antídoto antidote
antihistamina antihistamine
antihistamínico
antihistaminic
antipático unpleasant,
disagreeable
año year; **el — pasado**
last year; **tener... —s** to
be . . . years old
apagar la luz to turn off the
light
aparato device, appliance,
machine; — **intrauterino**
intrauterine device
apariencia appearance
apartamento apartment
apéndice *m* appendix
apetito appetite
apio celery
aplicaciones calientes *f pl*
hot compresses
aplicar to apply
aprender (a) to learn (to)
apretar to press, squeeze
apropiado appropriate

apuñalar to knife, stab
aquí here; **por —** around
here
arreglarse to arrange, work
out, fix
arriba above, up
arroz *m* rice
articulación *f* joint
artista *mf* artist
asegurar to assure
así so, thus, like this; **así así**
so-so
asignado assigned
asistenta assistant,
attendant, aide
asistente *m* assistant,
attendant, orderly
asma asthma
aspecto aspect, appearance
aspirar to inhale
aspirina aspirin
asumir to assume, take on
asustado frightened
ataque *m* attack; — **al**
corazón heart attack
atentar to attempt; — **el**
suicidio to attempt
suicide
atento attentive
atleta *mf* athlete
atontado bewildered,
stupified
atragantarse to choke
atrás behind, back
atrasado mentalmente
mentally retarded
atribuirse (a) to be
attributed to
atún *m* tuna
aturdido dazed
autor, -a author
autorización *f* authorization
averiguar to find out
avisar to warn, advise
ayer yesterday
ayuda help; enema
ayudar to help
azúcar *m* sugar

B
bacín *m* bedpan
bajarse (de) to go down, to
come down from
bajo short, low
balanceado balanced
banco bank
bañar to bathe someone;
—se to take a bath
baño bath
barbero barber
barbilla chin
barbiturato barbiturate
barbitúrico barbiturate
barras paralelas *f pl*
parallel bars
barriga belly
bastante enough, sufficient
bastón *m* cane, walking
stick
bata bathrobe
bazo spleen
beber to drink
bebida alcohólica alcoholic
drink
beneficioso beneficial
biberón *m* baby's bottle
bicúspide *m* bicuspid
bien well
bienestar *m* well-being
bifocales *m pl* bifocals
biología biology
bistec *m* beefsteak
bizcocho biscuit
blanco white
blando bland
boca mouth; — **abajo** on
one's stomach; — **arriba**
on one's back
bolsa de aguas bag of
waters
borracho *n* drunkard; *a*
drunk
borroso blurred
botar to throw away
botella bottle
brazo arm
bróculi *m* broccoli

bronquios *m pl* bronchial tubes
bronquitis *f* bronchitis
bueno good
buscar to look for

C

cabello hair
cabestrillo sling
cabeza head
cachete *m* cheek
cada each; every
cadera hip
caer to fall; **—se** to fall down, slip
café *m* coffee
cafetería cafeteria
cajero cashier
calambre *m* cramp
cálculo stone
calentura fever
caliente warm, hot
calmante *m* tranquilizer
calmarse to calm down
calor *m* heat; **tener —** to be warm
calle *f* street
cama bed
cámara cavity, chamber
camarera waitress
camarero waiter
camarones *m pl* shrimp
cambiar to change
cambio change; **en —** on the other hand
camilla stretcher; **llevar en —** to carry on a stretcher
camillero stretcher-bearer
caminar to walk
camisa shirt
cáncer *m* cancer
cangrejo crab
cansado tired
cansarse to become tired
cantidad *f* quantity
cápsula capsule
cardiólogo, -a cardiologist
cariado decayed

carie *f* tooth decay, cavity
carne *f* meat
carnicero butcher
carpintero carpenter
carta letter
cartero mailman
casa house; **en —** at home
casado married
caso case; **en todo —** in any case
cataratas *f pl* cataracts
catarro head cold; **tener —** to have a cold
catéter *m* catheter
causa cause; **a — de** because of
cebolla onion
ceja eyebrow
cepillarse los dientes to brush one's teeth
cepillo brush; **— de dientes** toothbrush
cereal *m* cereal
cerebro brain
cereza cherry
cerrado closed
cerrar to close
cerveza beer
cerviz *f* cervix
ciego blind
cielo de la boca roof of the mouth
cierto certain; **es —** it is certain; **por —** as a matter of fact
cigarrillo cigarette
cintura waist
ciruela plum; **— pasa** prune
cirugía surgery
cirujano, -a surgeon
cita appointment, date
ciudad *f* city
clavícula collar bone
clínica clinic
cocaína cocaine
cocer to cook
cocina kitchen
cocinar to cook

codeína codeine
codo elbow
coito coitus
cojo lame
colado strained
colesterol *m* cholesterol
cólico colic
coliflor *f* cauliflower
colmillo eyetooth
colon *m* colon
columna vertebral vertebral column
coma *m* coma
comer to eat; **dar de —** to feed
comida food
como as, like
¿cómo? how?; **¿cómo no?** of course
cómodo comfortable
compañía company; **— de seguro** insurance company
competente competent
complicación *f* complication
comportamiento behavior, bearing
comprender to understand
con with; **— respecto a** with respect to, regarding
condición *f* condition
condón *m* condom
conducto biliar bile duct
conductor *m* driver
confinar en una institución to confine in an institution
confuso confused, confusing
conjunto set
conmigo with me
conocimiento knowledge
consecuencia consequence
conseguir to obtain
consejero counselor
consejo advice, counsel
constante constant
consulta consultation; advice

consultar to consult
consultorio doctor's office
contacto contact
contaminación f
contamination
contento content
contracción f contraction
contracepción f
contraception
control m control
conveniente convenient
convulsión f convulsion
corazón m heart
cordero lamb
cordón umbilical m
umbilical cord
corea chorea
corona crown
correctamente correctly
correcto correct
correr to run; **— el riesgo**
to run the risk
cortar to cut; **—se** cut
oneself
cosa thing
costar to cost
costilla rib
cráneo skull
creer to believe
crema cream; **— de**
cacahuete peanut butter;
— vaginal vaginal cream
criatura infant
criminal m criminal
¿cuál? which?; what?
cualquier any
cuando when
¿cuándo? when?
¿cuánto? how much?; **¿—s?**
how many?
cuanto antes as soon as
possible
cuarto room; **— doble**
double room; **— múltiple**
ward; **— privado** private
room
cubrir to cover
cuchara spoon

cucharada spoonful
cuchillo knife
cuello neck
cuello uterino cervix
cuero cabelludo scalp
cuerpo body
cuidado care; **con —**
carefully; **— intensivo**
intensive care; **— prenatal**
prenatal care; **tener —** to
be careful
cuidar to care for, take care
of
cuñado, -a brother-in-law,
sister-in-law
cura m priest; f cure
curar to cure

CH

cheque m check
chequeo checkup
chichón m lump
chocolate m chocolate
choque nervioso m
nervous shock

D

daño hurt, harm; **hacerse**
— to hurt oneself
dar to give; **— a luz** to give
birth
de of, from; **— veras,**
— verdad truly, really,
indeed
deber m duty
deber to owe, must, should
débil weak
decidir to decide
decir to say, tell
decisión f decision; **tomar**
una — to make a decision
dedo finger; **— anular** ring
finger; **— del pie** toe;
— índice index finger;
— medio middle finger;
— meñique little finger;
— pulgar thumb
defecto congénito
congenital defect

defecto de nacimiento
birth defect
defender to defend
dejar to leave; **— de** to
stop, cease; **— en paz** to
leave (one) alone
del (de + **el)** of the
delgado thin, slender
demasiado too much; **—s**
too many
dentadura denture;
— completa full denture;
— parcial partial denture;
— postiza false teeth
dental dental
dentista mf dentist
dentro (de) inside of; **por —**
within
Departamento de
Seguridad Social
Department of Social
Security
dependiente, -a n clerk; a
dependent
deprimido depressed
derecho right, right side; **a**
la derecha to the right
desarrollo development
desayunarse to have
breakfast
desayuno breakfast; **tomar**
el — to have breakfast
descansar to rest
descanso rest
descubrir to discover
desde from, since
desear to desire, want
desintoxicación f
detoxification
desintoxicar to detoxicate
desmayarse to faint
desnutrición f malnutrition
despacio slowly
despertar to wake someone
up; **—se** to awaken
despierto awake
después (de) after
determinar to determine

detrás de behind

día *m* day; **al —** per day

diabético diabetic

diabetis *f* diabetes

diafragma *m* diaphragm

diagnóstico diagnosis

diarrea diarrhea

diciembre *m* December

diente *m* tooth; **— cariado** decayed tooth; **— de leche** milk tooth

dieta diet; **seguir una —** to follow a diet

diferente different

difícil difficult

dificultad *f* difficulty

difteria diphtheria

digerido digested

digerir to digest

digestión *f* digestion

digestivo digestive; **sistema —** *m* digestive system

dilatación *f* dilation; **— del cuello de la matriz** dilation of the cervix

diligente diligent

dinero money

dirección *f* direction; address

dirigir direct; **—se (a)** to go toward, direct oneself to

discutir to discuss

disentería dysentery

dislexia dyslexia

divertirse to have fun, enjoy oneself

divorciado divorced

doblar to bend, turn

doctor, -a doctor

dolor *m* pain; **— de cabeza** headache; **— del oído** earache; **—es del parto** labor pains; **tener —** to be in pain

domingo Sunday

donde where

¿dónde? where?; **¿a —?** to where?; **¿de —?** from where?

dormido asleep, sleeping

dormir to sleep; **—se** to fall asleep

dorso spine, back; **— de la mano** back of the hand

dosis excesiva *f* overdose

droga drug

ducha shower, douche

duda doubt, **sin —** without a doubt, undoubtedly

dudar to doubt

dudoso doubtful

durante during

durar to last

duro hard

E

eczema eczema

echar to throw

efecto secundario side effect

eficaz (*pl* **eficaces**) efficient

ejercer to exercise

ejercicio exercise; **hacer los —s** to exercise

electricista *mf* electrician

eliminar to eliminate

embarazada pregnant

embarazarse to become pregnant

embarazo pregnancy

emergencia emergency

emocional emotional

empastar to fill a tooth, do a filling

empaste *m* filling

empeine *m* instep

empeorar to worsen, become worse

empleo employment, work, job

empujar to push

en in, on; **— cuanto a** as for

encargarse (de) to take charge of

encender la luz to turn on the light

encía gum

encinta pregnant

encontrar to find, meet

enema enema

enero January

enfermarse to become sick

enfermedad *f* sickness; **— contagiosa** contagious disease; **— transmisible** communicable disease; **— venérea** venereal disease

enfermero, -a nurse

enfermo sick

enfrentarse (con) to face, confront

enfrente (de) in front of

enjuagarse to rinse

enojado angry

enriquecido enriched

ensuciar to dirty

entonces then

entrar to enter

entre among, between

entrepiernas *f pl* crotch

envenenarse to be poisoned

enyesar to put in a cast

epilepsia epilepsy

eructar to belch; **tener —s** to have gas, to belch

eructo belch

escaldadura diaper rash

escalera stairs, staircase; **— abajo** downstairs; **— arriba** upstairs

escalofrío chill

escaparse to escape

escápula shoulder blade

escarlatina scarlet fever

escoger to choose

escribir to write

escudo shield

escuela school

escupir to spit

esencial essential

esmalte *m* polish; enamel

espalda back
español *n m* Spanish (language); Spaniard; *a* Spanish
espárrago asparagus
especia spice
especial special
especialista *mf* specialist
especializarse to specialize
específico specific
espejuelos *m pl* eyeglasses
esperar to wait, to hope
esperma sperm, semen
espinaca spinach
espinilla shin
espiral *f* spiral
esplín *m* spleen
esposo husband; **-a** wife
esqueleto skeleton
estado state; **— civil** marital status; **— de salud** state of health
estar to be; **— a favor de** to be in favor of; **— de acuerdo con** to agree with; **— de pie** to be standing; **— en estado** to be pregnant; **— seguro de** to be sure of
esterilización *f* sterilization
esterilizar to sterilize
esternón *m* breastbone
estómago stomach
estornudar to sneeze
estrenuo strenuous
estreñido constipated
estreñimiento constipation
estudiar to study
etiqueta label
evitar to avoid
examen *m* test
excepción *f* exception; **con — de** except for
exceso excess
exigente demanding
existir to exist
experimentar to experience
explicación *f* explanation
expresar to express

extracción *f* extraction
extraer to extract
extraño strange
extremidad *f* extremity

F
fábrica factory
fácil easy
fácilmente easily
factor *m* factor
familia family
familiar *n mf* relative, family member; *a* familiar
familiarizarse (con) to become familiar with
farmacéutico pharmacist
farmacia pharmacy
favor *m* favor; **— de + inf** please; **por —** please
febrero February
feo ugly
fértil fertile
feto fetus
fibroma *m* fibroma
fiebre *f* fever; **— amarilla** yellow fever; **— de heno** hay fever; **— reumática** rheumatic fever
fin *m* end; **por —** finally
firmar to sign
físico physical
fisioterapia physical therapy
flaco thin, slender, skinny
flema phlegm
flexible flexible
fluido fluid
flujo de sangre discharge of blood
forceps *m* forceps
forma form
fórmula formula
formulario form, application
fosas nasales *f pl* nostrils
foto *f* photograph; **sacar —s** to take pictures
fracturar to fracture
frecuencia frequency; **con —** frequently

frecuentemente frequently
frente *f* forehead
fresa strawberry
frijol *m* bean
frío cold; **tener —** to be cold
fruta fruit
fuerte strong
fumar to smoke
función *f* function
funcionar to function, work; **— mal** to malfunction

G
gafas *f pl* eyeglasses; **— de sol** sunglasses
galleta cracker, biscuit
ganar to win
gangrena gangrene
garganta throat
gárgara gargling; **hacer —s** to gargle
gas *m* gas
gasto expense, cost
gastritis *m* gastritis
gastrointestinal gastrointestinal
gelatina gelatin
gemelo twin
ginecólogo, -a gynecologist
glaucoma *m* glaucoma
globo del ojo eyeball
gonorrea gonorrhea
gordo fat
gorro cervical cervical cap
gota drop
gracias thank you; **¡— a Dios!** thank God!
gradual gradual
grande large, big; great
grasa grease, fat
grasoso greasy, fatty
gratis free, gratis
grave serious, grave
guapo handsome, pretty
guisante *m* pea
gustar to like, please; to be pleasing to
(mucho) gusto it's a pleasure

H

habichuela verde green bean
habilidad *f* ability
hábito habit
hablar to speak, talk
hacer to make, do
hacia toward
hambre *f* hunger; **tener —** to be hungry; **tener mucha —** to be very hungry
hamburguesa hamburger
hasta until
hay there is, there are
helado ice cream
hemorragia hemorrhage
hemorroides *m pl* hemorrhoids
hepatitis *f* hepatitis
hermano brother; **-a** sister
hermoso beautiful
heroína heroin
hierro iron
hígado liver
hija daughter
hijo son; **—s** children
hinchazón *m* swelling
hiperactivo hyperactive
hirviente boiling
histerectomía hysterectomy
hombre *m* man
hombro shoulder
hongo mushroom
hora hour; time; **¿qué — es?** what time is it?
hospital *m* hospital
hospitalizar to hospitalize
hoy today
huevo egg; **— duro** hard-boiled egg; **— frito** fried egg; **— pasado por agua** soft-boiled egg; **— revuelto** scrambled egg
húmedo moist, damp, wet

I

idea idea
idioma *m* language

impaciente impatient
impactado impacted
impedimento impediment
impertinente impertinent
impétigo impetigo
importante important
impulsar to impel
incisivo incisor
incluir to include; **—se** to be included
incómodo uncomfortable
incompetente incompetent
incomprensible incomprehensible
incubadora incubator
indicar to indicate
indigestión *f* indigestion
inferior inferior
inflamación *f* inflammation
inflamado inflamed
inflexible inflexible
influenza influenza, flu
información *f* information
ingeniero, -a engineer
inglés *n m* English (language); *a* English
inhalar to inhale
inmunización *f* immunization
inmunizar to immunize
inocular to inoculate
inquieto restless
insertar to insert
institución *f* institution
instrucción *f* instruction
insulina insulin
inteligente intelligent
interesado interested; **estar — en** to be interested in
intestino intestine
intravenoso intravenous
inútil useless
investigar to investigate
inyección *f* injection; **— intravenosa** intravenous injection
inyectar to inject
ir to go; **— a** + *inf* to be going to; **—se** to leave

irregular irregular
irresponsable irresponsible
irritación *f* irritation
irritado irritated
irritar to irritate
izquierdo left, left side; **a la izquierda** to the left

J

jabón *m* soap
jamón *m* ham
jaqueca headache
jarabe *m* syrup
joven *n mf* youth; *a* young
jueves *m* Thursday
jugo juice; **— de china, — de naranja** orange juice; **— de tomate** tomato juice; **— de toronja** grapefruit juice
julio July

L

labio lip
labor *f* labor
laboratorio laboratory
lado side
langosta lobster
lápiz (*pl* **lápices**) *m* pencil
laringitis *f* laryngitis
lástima *pity;* **¡qué —!** what a pity!
lavabo washbasin
lavado enema; **— vaginal** douche
lavaplatos *m* dishwasher
lavar to wash; **—se** to wash oneself
lavativa enema
lazo loop
lección *f* lesson
lectura reading
leche *f* milk; **— de magnesia** milk of magnesia
lechuga lettuce
leer to read
legumbre *f* vegetable
lengua tongue; language

lente *m* lens; **— de contacto** contact lens
lesión *f* lesion, injury
lesionarse to be injured
leucemia leukemia
levantar to raise, lift; **—se** to get up, arise
leve light, slight
ley *f* law
libro book
ligadura de los tubos tubal ligation
limitación *f* limitation
limitado limited
limón *m* lemon
limpiar to clean
limpieza cleaning
limpio clean
línea line
linimento liniment
líquido liquid
listo ready; **estar —** to be ready; **ser —** to be clever
loco insane, crazy
lo mismo the same
lo que that which
luego then, later
lunes *m* Monday
luz (*pl* **luces**) *f* light; **encender la —** to turn on the light

LL
llamada telefónica telephone call
llamar to call; **—se** to be called, named
llegar to arrive
llenar to fill
lleno full
llevar to carry; **— en camilla** to carry on a stretcher
llorar to cry

M
madre *f* mother
madrugada dawn

maestro, -a teacher
maíz *m* corn
mal badly
malaria malaria
malestar *m* ailment
maleta suitcase
maligno malignant
malo bad
maltrato de los niños child abuse
mamá mother, mommy
mamar to breast-feed
mamografía mammography
mandar to order, command
mandíbula jaw
manera way, manner; **de esta —** in this manner; **de ninguna —** in no way
mano *f* hand
manta blanket
mantequilla butter
manzana apple
mañana morning; tomorrow; **de la —** A.M.; **por la —** in the morning
máquina machine; **— ultrasónica** ultrasonic machine
mareado dizzy, seasick
mareo dizziness, seasickness; **tener —** to be dizzy, seasick
margarina margarine
marido husband
marihuana marijuana
mariscos *m pl* shellfish
martes *m* Tuesday
más more; **— o menos** more or less
masaje *m* massage
mastectomía mastectomy
masticar to chew
materia radioactiva radioactive material
maternidad *f* maternity
matriz *f* womb, matrix
mayo May
mayonesa mayonnaise
mayor older; **el/la —** the oldest

mecánico mechanic
medianoche *f* midnight
medicamento medicine, medication
médico physician, doctor
medio half; middle; **por — de** by means of
mediodía *m* noon; **al —** at noon
medir to measure
mejilla cheek
mejor better; **a lo —** maybe, perhaps; **es —** it is better
mejorarse to improve, get better
melocotón *m* peach
meningitis *f* meningitis
menor younger; **el/la menor** the youngest
menos less, least; **por lo —** at least
menstruación *f* menstruation
mentir to lie
mentón *m* chin
(a) menudo often
mes *m* month
mesa table
mescalina mescaline
meter to put in, to insert
método method; **— anticonceptivo** birth control method; **— de ritmo** rhythm method
miedo fear; **tener —** to be afraid
miembro member; penis
mientras while; **— tanto** in the meantime
miércoles *m* Wednesday
migraña migraine
mirar to look at
mismo same; **ahora —** right now
molestar to bother
molestia bother
molesto bothersome, bothered

momento moment
morir to die
mostrar to show
mover to move
muchacho boy; **-a** girl;
  —s children, boys
mucho much, many;
  muchas veces often
muela molar; **— del juicio**
  impactado impacted
  wisdom tooth
muerto dead
mujer *f* woman
muleta crutch
muñeca wrist
muslo thigh
muy very

N

nacer to be born
nacimiento birth
nada nothing; **de —** you're
  welcome
nadie no one
nalga buttock
naranja orange
narcótico narcotic
nariz *f* nose; **— tupida**
  stuffy nose
natalidad *f* birth
náuseas *f pl* nausea; **— del**
  embarazo morning
  sickness
necesario necessary
necesidad *f* necessity
necesitar to need
negocio business
nene, -a baby, infant
nervio nerve
nervioso nervous
neurólogo, -a neurologist
neutralizar to neutralize
ningún, ninguno none, not
  any
niño boy; **-a** girl; **—s**
  children, boys
no no, not; **— hay de qué**
  you're welcome
noche *f* night; **de la —**

P.M.; **por la —** in the
  evening
nombre *m* name
normal normal
notar to note, notice
noticia news; notice
notificar to notify
noviembre *m* November
novio boyfriend; **-a**
  girlfriend
nuca nape
nudillo knuckle
nudo knot, lump
nuera daughter-in-law
nuez de Adán *f* Adam's
  apple
número number
nutrición *f* nutrition

O

obstetricia obstetrics
obstétrico, -a obstetrician
obstruir el nervio to
  obstruct the nerve
obvio obvious
octubre *m* October
ocupado busy, occupied
ocurrir to occur, happen
oficial *m* official
oficina office
ofrecer to offer
oftalmólogo, -a
  ophthalmologist
oído ear, hearing
ojo *eye*
olvidar to forget, leave
  behind; **—se (de)** to forget
  (about)
ombligo navel
omóplato shoulder blade
operación *f* operation
operar to operate
opinión *f* opinion
óptico optician
optometrista *mf* optometrist
oral oral; **por vía —** to be
  taken orally
orden *m* order, harmony; *f*
  order, command

oreja ear, outer ear
órgano organ; **—s**
  genitales genital organs
orina urine
ortopédico, -a orthopedist
ostra oyster
otro other, another; **otra**
  vez again
ovario ovary
oxígeno oxygen

P

paciencia patience
paciente *mf* patient
padecer to suffer, be
  afflicted with
padre *m* father; **—s**
  parents
pagar to pay
palabra word
paladar *m* palate
pálido pale
palma de la mano palm of
  the hand
palpitación *f* palpitation
paludismo malaria
pan *m* bread; **— blanco**
  white bread; **— de centeno**
  rye bread; **— de trigo**
  entero whole wheat bread
páncreas *m* pancreas
pantorrilla calf
pañal *m* diaper;
  — desechable disposable
  diaper; **— de tela** cloth
  diaper
papa potato; **— asada**
  baked potato; **— frita** fried
  potato
papá *m* father, daddy
paperas *f pl* mumps
paquete *m* package
par *m* pair, couple; **un — de**
  a couple of
para for; **— que** so that;
  ¿— qué? what for?
parado standing
parálisis *m* paralysis; **—**
  cerebral cerebral palsy

paralizado paralyzed

pararse to stop; to stand up

parecer to seem

pariente, -a *n* relative

párpado eyelid

parte *f* part

partera midwife

participar to participate

particular particular

partir to split, divide; depart;
a — de from, starting from

parto childbirth; **—
múltiple** multiple
childbirth; **— natural**
natural childbirth; **—
prematuro** premature
childbirth

pasado past; **el año —** last
year; **— mañana** the day
after tomorrow

pasar to happen; to pass; to
enter; **¿Qué pasa?** What's
the matter?

paso preparativo
preparatory step

pastel *m* pie, cake

pastilla pill; **— para dormir**
sleeping pill

pecho breast, chest; **dar el
—** to breast-feed

pediatra *mf* pediatrician

peligroso dangerous

pelo hair

pelvis *f* pelvis

pene *m* penis

penetrante penetrating

penetrar to penetrate

penicilina penicillin

pensar to think; **— +** *inf*
to intend to; **— de** to think
about

peor worse

pepinillo pickle

pepino cucumber

pera pear

perder to lose; **— el
conocimiento** to lose
consciousness

perdonar to pardon

periódico newspaper

período period

permiso permission; **con su
—** with your permission,
excuse me

permitir to permit

pero but

personal personal

pesadilla nightmare

pesar to weigh

pescado fish

peso weight; **aumentar de
—** to gain weight; **perder
—** to lose weight

pestaña eyelash

pezón *m* nipple; **— de
biberón** nipple on baby's
bottle

pie *m* foot; **al — de la letra**
to the letter, verbatim

piedra stone; **— biliar**
gallstone; **— nefrítica**
kidney stone

piel *f* skin

pielograma intravenoso *m*
intravenous pyelogram

pierna leg

pijamas *f pl* pajamas

píldora pill; **— para dormir**
sleeping pill

pimienta pepper

piorrea pyorrhea

piso floor

pistola pistol

planta del pie sole of the
foot

plátano plantain, banana

pluma pen

poco little; **— a —** little by
little; **—s** few; **un —** a
little

poder to be able; **puede ser**
it may be

policía *m* policeman; *f*
police

poliomielitis *f* poliomyelitis

pollo chicken

poner to put; **— en
cabestrillo** to put in a

sling; **— una inyección** to
give an injection; **—se +** *adj*
to become; **—se borroso**
to become blurred; **—se de
pie** to stand; **—se la ropa**
to put on one's clothing

por for; by; because of; **— sí
mismo** by one's self; **—
supuesto** of course

porque because

¿por qué? why?

posible possible

posiblemente possibly

postre *m* dessert

práctica practice

precaucionarse to take
precautions

preferible preferable

preferiblemente preferably

preferir to prefer

pregunta question; **hacer
una —** to ask a question

preguntar to ask, question

preñada pregnant

preocupado worried

preocuparse to worry

preparar to prepare

presión *f* pressure; **— alta**
high blood pressure;
— arterial blood pressure;
— baja low blood
pressure; **tomar la —** to
take the blood pressure

prestar to lend

primero first

primo, -a cousin

prisa *f* hurry; **tener —** to
be in a hurry

privado private

probar to test, try, prove

problema *m* problem

procedimiento procedure

producido (por) produced
by

producir to produce

profesión *f* profession

profesor, -a professor

profiláctico prophylactic

profundamente profoundly

pronóstico prognosis, forecast

pronto soon; **lo más — posible** as soon as possible

propósito purpose; **a —** by the way; on purpose

protección *f* protection

proteger to protect

proteína protein

próximo next

prueba test; **— del embarazo** pregnancy test

psicólogo, -a psychologist

psiquíatra *mf* psychiatrist

psiquiatría psychiatry

pudín *m* pudding

puente *m* bridge

puerco pork

puerta door

pulgar *m* thumb

pulmón *m* lung

pulmonía pneumonia

pulso pulse; **registrar el —** to take the pulse

punto point

puño fist; **hacer un —** to make a fist

pupila pupil

Q

que that; **hay —** it is necessary; **tener —** to have to

¿qué? what?

quedar to have left over; to remain; **—se** to stay, remain; **—se con** to keep

quejarse (de) to complain (about)

quemadura burn

quemante burning

quemar to burn; **—se** to burn oneself

querer to want, wish; love

queso cheese; **— crema** cream cheese

quien who, whom

¿quién? who?, whom?; **¿de —?** whose?

quieto still, quiet

quijada jaw

quiste *m* cyst

quitar to take away; **—se** to remove, take off

quizá(s) maybe, perhaps

R

rábano radish

radioactivo radioactive

radiografía X-ray; **hacer una —** to take an X-ray

raíz (*pl* **raíces**) *f* root

rápidamente quickly

rápido fast

raquitis *m* rickets

rascarse to scratch oneself

razón *f* reason; **tener —** to be right

reacción *f* reaction; **— alérgica** allergic reaction

realidad *f* reality; **en —** in reality

recepcionista *mf* receptionist

receta prescription

recetar to precribe

recibir to receive

recoger to pick up

reconocimiento médico physical exam

recordar to remember

recto straight

recuperar to recuperate

recurrir (a) to resort to

referirse to refer

regalo gift

registrar el pulso to take the pulse

regla rule; menstrual period

reírse (de) to laugh (at)

relaciones sexuales *f pl* sexual relations

relajarse to relax

relativamente relatively

remolacha beet

requerir to require

requesón *m* cottage cheese

(carne de) res *f* beef

resfriado cold

resistencia resistance

respiración *f* respiration; **— artificial** artificial respiration; **— boca a boca** mouth-to-mouth resuscitation

respirar to breathe

respiratorio respiratory

responder to respond, answer

responsabilidad *f* responsibility

responsable responsible

resucitar to resuscitate

resultado result

retirada withdrawal

rico rich

riesgo risk

riñón *m* kidney

rodilla knee

romper to break

ronquera hoarseness

ropa clothing; **— interior** underwear

rosbif *m* roast beef

rótula patella

rubéola German measles

ruido noise

S

sacar to remove, take out

sacarina saccharin

sal *f* salt

sala room; **— de espera** waiting room; **— de partos** delivery room; **— de recuperación** recovery room

salir to leave; **— bien** to turn out well; **— mal** to turn out badly

saliva saliva

salmón *m* salmon

salpullido rash

sangre *f* blood
sangrar to bleed
sarampión *m* measles
sardina sardine
sección cesárea *f*
caesarean section
seco dry
seguido continuously
según according to
seguridad *f* safety; **con —**
safely
semana week; **— pasada**
last week; **— que viene**
next week
sensación *f* sensation
señal *f* sign, signal
señalar to signal
separado separated
ser to be; **— cuestión de**
to be a question of;
— humano human being
serio serious
servicio service
servir to serve
severo severe
sexual sexual
si if; **— no** if not
sí yes
siempre always
simpático likable, nice
sin without; **— duda**
undoubtedly; **— embargo**
nevertheless
sistema *m* system;
— circulatorio circulatory
system; **— digestivo**
digestive system;
— nervioso nervous
system; **— respiratorio**
respiratory system
sobre over, above, on top
of; **— todo** above all
sobrio sober
soda soda
solicitar to solicit, ask for
sólido solid
soltero single, unmarried
solución *f* solution
sonda catheter

sopa soup
sordo deaf
sospechar to suspect
substancia radioactiva
radioactive substance
suceder to happen
sucio dirty
suficiente sufficient
sufrir (de) to suffer (from)
suicidio suicide; **atentar el**
— to attempt suicide
sulfato de bario barium
sulfate

T

tableta tablet
tal such, such as
taladrar to drill
taladro drill
talco talcum
talón *m* heel
tamaño size
tambalear to stagger
también also, too
tampoco not. . .either,
neither
tan so, as
tanto as much, so much; **—s**
as many
tarde *f* afternoon; *a* late;
de la — P.M.; **por la —** in
the afternoon
taza cup
té *m* tea
técnico technician
telefónico *a* telephone,
phone
teléfono telephone
televisión *f* television
temperatura temperature
temprano early
terapeuta *mf* therapist
terapia física physical
therapy
terapista *mf* therapist; **—**
físico physical therapist
terminar to finish, end
ternera veal
testículo testicle

tétano tetanus
tía aunt
tiempo time; weather; **al**
mismo — at the same
time; **¿cuanto — hace?**
how long has it been?; **hace**
buen — the weather is
good; **hace mucho —** it
has been a long time; **¿que**
— hace? what is the
weather like?
tifoidea typhoid
timbre *m* bell
tinta ink; **— de yodo**
tincture of iodine
tío uncle
tipo type, kind
tirar (de) to pull
toalla towel
tobillo ankle
tocar to touch
tocino bacon
todavía still, yet
todo every; **—s** all; **—s los**
días every day
tolerante tolerant
tomar to take; **— medidas**
to take measures
tomate *m* tomato
tontería foolishness
tórax *m* thorax
torcedura sprain
torcer to twist, turn, sprain
torniquete *m* tourniquet
toronja grapefruit
torta cake
tortilla omelette
tos *f* cough; **— ferina**
whooping cough
toser to cough
toxemia toxemia
trabajador *m* worker
trabajar to work
trabajo work
tradicional traditional
traer to bring
tragar to swallow
tranquilizante *m*
tranquilizer

tranquilo calm, tranquil
transmisor ultrasonido *m* ultrasound transmitter
transmitir to transmit
tratamiento treatment
tratar (de) to try to
través: a — de through; by means of
triste sad
tuberculosis *f* tuberculosis
tubo pipe; tube
tumor *m* tumor
turno turn

U

úlcera ulcer
último last
ungüento ointment
único only; unique
uña nail
urinálisis *m* urinalysis
usar to use
útero uterus

V

vacío empty
vagina vagina
valiente brave
variado varied
vasectomía vasectomy
vasija receptacle, container
vaso drinking glass
vecino *n* neighbor; *a* neighboring

vegetal *m* vegetable
vejiga bladder
velar to watch over
venda bandage
vendaje *m* bandages, dressing
vender to sell
veneno poison
venir to come
ventaja advantage
ventana window
ver to see
verdad *f* truth; **de —** really, truly, indeed
verduras *f pl* greens
vértigo dizziness
vesícula biliar gallbladder
vestirse to dress oneself, to get dressed
vez (*pl* **veces**) *f* time; **a —s** at times; sometimes; **muchas —s** many times; **pocas —s** few times, seldom; **una —** one time, once
víctima victim
vientre *m* womb, abdomen
viernes *m* Friday
vinagre *m* vinegar
vínculo link
vino wine
violación *f* rape; violation
violar to rape, violate
viruela smallpox; **—s locas** chicken pox

virus *m* virus
visión *f* vision
visita visit
visitar to visit
vista sight, vision; **tener buena —** to have good vision
vitamina vitamin
viudo, -a widower, widow
vivir to live
volar to fly
volver to return
vomitar to vomit
vómito vomit, vomiting; **—s del embarazo** morning sickness

Y

y and
ya already; **— no** no longer; **— que** since, inasmuch as
yema del huevo egg yolk
yerno son-in-law
yeso plaster cast; **poner en —** to put in a cast
yodo iodine

Z

zanahoria carrot
zapatilla slipper
zapato shoe

English to Spanish

A

to abandon abandonar
abdomen abdomen *m*
ability habilidad *f*
to be able poder
abnormality anormalidad *f*
abortion aborto, aborto provocado; **therapeutic —** aborto terapéutico
above arriba; sobre, encima de
to abstain abstener(se)
to accept aceptar
accident accidente *m*
according to según
acidity acidez *f*
activity actividad *f*
actor actor *m*
actress actriz *f*
Adam's apple nuez de Adán *f*
addict adicto; **addicted to** adicto a
additional adicional
to adopt adoptar
adult adulto
advantage ventaja
advice consejo
to advise aconsejar
after después (de)
afternoon tarde *f*
aggressive agresivo
to agree (with) estar de acuerdo (con)

ahead adelante
ailment malestar *m*
air aire *m*; **— conditioning** aire acondicionado
alcohol alcohol *m*
alcoholic alcohólico; **— drink** bebida alcohólica
alcoholism alcoholismo
all todos
allergic alérgico; **— reaction** reacción alérgica
allergy alergia
already ya
also también
alternative alternativa
always siempre
ambulance ambulancia
among entre
amphetamine anfetamina
to amputate amputar
analgesic analgésico
analysis análisis *m*; **to do an —** hacer un análisis
to analyze analizar
anatomy anatomía
and y
anemia anemia
anesthesia anestesia; **caudal —** anestesia caudal; **general —** anestesia general; **local —** anestesia local
anesthesiologist anestesiólogo, -a

anesthetic anestético
to anesthetize anestesiar
angry enojado
ankle tobillo
another otro
antacid antiácido
antibiotic antibiótico
antidote antídoto
antihistamine antihistamina
antihistaminic antihistamínico
anus ano
any alguno; cualquier
apartment apartamento
appearance apariencia, aspecto
appendix apéndice *m*
appetite apetito
apple manzana
appliance aparato
to apply (to oneself) aplicar(se)
appointment cita
to approach acercar(se) a
appropriate apropiado
apricot albaricoque *m*
April abril *m*
arm brazo
to arrange arreglar
to arrive llegar
artist artista *mf*
as tan; como; **— for** en cuanto a
to ask preguntar; **to — for** solicitar

asleep dormido
asparagus espárrago
aspect aspecto
aspirin aspirina
assigned asignado
assistant asistente, -a
to assume asumir
to assure asegurar
asthma asma
at a
athlete atleta *mf*
attack ataque *m;* **heart —**
 ataque al corazón
attendant asistente, -a
attentive atento
attitude actitud *f*
attorney abogado
August agosto
aunt tía
author autor, -a
authorization autorización *f*
to avoid evitar
awake despierto
to awaken (someone)
 despertar; **to wake up**
 despertarse

B

baby nene, -a; niño, -a
back (behind) *prep* atrás; *n*
 espalda; **on one's —** boca
 arriba
bacon tocino
bad malo
badly mal
balanced balanceado
banana banana, plátano
bandage venda
bank banco
barber barbero
barbiturate barbiturato,
 barbitúrico
barium sulfate sulfato de
 bario
bath baño
to bathe bañar; **to take a**
 bath bañarse
bathrobe bata
to be estar; ser

bean frijol *m;* **green —**
 habichuela verde
beautiful hermoso
because porque; **— of** a
 causa de
to become ponerse
bed cama; **to go to —**
 acostarse; **to put to —**
 acostar
bedpan bacín *m*
beef carne de res *f*
beefsteak bistec *m*
beer cerveza
beet remolacha
before antes (de)
to begin comenzar, empezar
behavior comportamiento
behind atrás, detrás de
belch eructo
to belch eructar, tener
 eructos
to believe creer, pensar
bell timbre *m*
belly barriga
to bend doblar
beneficial beneficioso
besides además de
better mejor; **to get —**
 mejorar(se)
between entre
bewildered atontado
bicuspid bicúspide *m*
bifocals bifocales *m pl*
big grande
bile duct conducto biliar
biology biología
birth nacimiento; natalidad;
 to give — dar a luz
biscuit bizcocho, galleta
bitter agrio
bladder vejiga
bland blando
blanket manta
to bleed sangrar
blind ciego
blood sangre *f*
blurred borroso; **to**
 become — ponerse borroso

body cuerpo
boiling hirviente
book libro
bored, boring aburrido
to be born nacer
bother molestia
to bother molestar
bothersome molesto
bottle botella; **baby's —**
 biberón *m*
boy muchacho
boyfriend novio
brain cerebro
brave valiente
bread pan *m;* **rye —** pan
 de centeno; **white —** pan
 blanco; **whole wheat —**
 pan de trigo entero
to break romper
breakfast desayuno; **to**
 have — tomar el
 desayuno, desayunar(se)
breast pecho
breastbone esternón *m*
to breast-feed dar el pecho,
 mamar
to breathe respirar
bridge puente *m*
to bring traer
broccoli brócoli *m*
bronchial tubes bronquios
 m pl
bronchitis bronquitis *f*
brother hermano
brother-in-law cuñado
brush cepillo; **toothbrush**
 cepillo de dientes
to brush cepillar(se)
burn quemadura
to burn quemar; **to —**
 oneself quemarse
burning quemante
business negocio
busy ocupado
but pero
butcher carnicero
butter mantequilla
buttock nalga

C

caesarean section sección cesárea *f*
cafeteria cafetería
cake torta
calf pantorrilla
to call llamar; **to be called** llamarse
calm tranquilo
to calm down calmar(se)
cancer cáncer *m*
cane bastón *m*
capsule cápsula
cardiologist cardiólogo, -a
care cuidado; **intensive —** cuidado intensivo; **prenatal —** cuidado prenatal
to care for cuidar (a)
carefully con cuidado, cuidadosamente
carpenter carpintero
carrot zanahoria
to carry llevar; **— on a stretcher** llevar en camilla
case caso; **in any —** en todo caso
cashier cajero
cast yeso; **to put in a —** enyesar, poner en yeso
cataracts cataratas
catheter catéter *m*, sonda
cauliflower coliflor *f*
cause causa
cavity carie *f*
celery apio
cereal cereal *m*
cerebral palsy parálisis cerebral *m*
certain cierto
cervical cap gorro cervical
cervix cerviz *f*, cuello uterino
change cambio
to change cambiar
check cheque *m*
checkup chequeo
cheek cachete *m*, mejilla
cheese queso; **cream —** queso crema
cherry cereza

to chew masticar
chicken pollo
chicken pox viruelas locas
child niño, -a; **child abuse** maltrato de los niños
childbirth parto; **multiple —** parto múltiple; **natural —** parto natural; **premature —** parto prematuro
chill escalofrío
chin barbilla, mentón *m*
chocolate chocolate *m*
to choke atragantar(se)
cholesterol colesterol *m*
to choose escoger
chorea corea
cigarette cigarrillo
city ciudad *f*
clam almeja
clean limpio
to clean limpiar
cleaning limpieza
clerk dependiente, -a
clinic clínica
closed cerrado
clothing ropa
cocaine cocaína
codeine codeína
coffee café *m*
coitus coito
cold frío; catarro, resfriado; **to be —** tener frío; **to have a —** tener catarro, tener un resfriado
colic cólico
collar bone clavícula
colon colon *m*
coma coma *m*
to come venir
comfortable cómodo
company compañía; **insurance —** compañía de seguro
competent competente
to complain quejar(se)
complication complicación *f*
(hot) compresses aplicaciones calientes *f pl*

condition condición *f*
condom condón *m*
to confine in an institution confinar en una institución
to confront enfrentar(se) con
confused, confusing confuso
consequence consecuencia
constant constante
constipated estreñido
constipation estreñimiento
to consult consultar
consultation consulta
contact contacto
contamination contaminación *f*
content contento
continuously continuamente, seguido
contraception contracepción *f*
contraceptive anticonceptivo
contraction contracción *f*
control control *m*
convenient conveniente
convulsion convulsión *f*
to cook cocer, cocinar
corn maíz *m*
correct correcto
correctly correctamente
cost gasto
to cost costar
cough tos *f*
to cough toser
counselor consejero
couple par *m;* **a — of** un par de
(of) course por supuesto
cousin primo, -a
to cover cubrir
crab cangrejo
cracker galleta
cramp calambre *m*
crazy loco
criminal criminal
crotch entrepiernas *f pl*
crown corona

crutch muleta
to cry llorar
cucumber pepino
cup taza
cure cura *f*
to cure curar
to cut cortar; **— oneself** cortarse
cyst quiste *m*

D
damp húmedo
dangerous peligroso
daughter hija
daughter-in-law nuera
dawn madrugada
day día *m;* **the — after tomorrow** pasado mañana; **the — before yesterday** anteayer
dazed aturdido
dead muerto
deaf sordo
(tooth) decay carie *f*
decayed cariado
December diciembre *m*
to decide decidir
decision decisión *f;* **to make a —** tomar una decisión
defect defecto; **birth —** defecto de nacimiento; **congenital —** defecto congénito
to defend defender
delivery room sala de partos
demanding exigente
dental dental
dentist dentista *mf*
denture dentadura; **full —** dentadura completa; **partial —** dentadura parcial
Department of Social Security Departamento de Seguridad Social
dependent dependiente
depressed deprimido
to desire desear, querer

dessert postre *m*
to determine determinar
to detoxicate desintoxicar
detoxification desintoxicación *f*
development desarrollo
device aparato; **intrauterine —** aparato intrauterino
diabetes diabetis *f*
diabetic diabético
diagnosis diagnóstico
diaper pañal *m;* **cloth —** pañal de tela; **— rash** escaldadura; **disposable —** pañal desechable
diaphragm diafragma *m*
diarrhea diarrea
to die morir
diet dieta; **to follow a —** seguir una dieta
different diferente
difficult difícil
difficulty dificultad *f*
to digest digerir
digested digerido
digestion digestión *f*
digestive digestivo; **— system** sistema digestivo *m*
dilation of the cervix dilatación del cuello de la matriz *f*
diligent diligente
diphtheria difteria
to direct oneself to dirigirse a
direction dirección *f*
dirty sucio
to dirty ensuciar
discharge flujo
to discover descubrir
to discuss discutir
disease enfermedad *f;* **communicable —** enfermedad transmisible; **contagious —** enfermedad contagiosa; **venereal —** enfermedad venérea

dishwasher lavaplatos *m*
divorced divorciado
dizziness mareo, vértigo
dizzy mareado; **to be —** tener mareo, estar mareado
to do hacer
doctor doctor, -a
door puerta
doubt duda; **without a —** sin duda
to doubt dudar
doubtful dudoso
douche ducha, lavado vaginal
down abajo; **to go —** bajar(se)
to dress (someone) vestir; **to get dressed** vestirse
dressing vendaje *m*
drill taladro
to drill taladrar
to drink beber
driver conductor *m*
drop gota
to drown ahogar(se)
drug droga
drunk borracho
dry seco
during durante
duty deber *m*
dysentery disentería
dyslexia dislexia

E
each cada
ear oído, oreja
earache dolor del oído *m*
early temprano
easily fácilmente
easy fácil
to eat comer
eczema eczema
efficient eficaz
egg huevo; **fried —** huevo frito; **hard-boiled —** huevo duro; **soft-boiled —** huevo pasado por agua; **scrambled —** huevo revuelto

egg yolk yema del huevo
elbow codo
elderly anciano, viejo
electrician electricista *mf*
to eliminate eliminar
emergency emergencia
emotional emocional
employment empleo, trabajo
empty vacío
enamel esmalte *m*
end fin *m*
enema ayuda, enema, lavado, lavativa
engineer ingeniero, -a
English inglés
to enjoy oneself divertirse
enough bastante
enriched enriquecido
to enter entrar, pasar
environment ambiente *m*
epilepsy epilepsia
to escape escapar(se)
essential esencial
every cada; todo
except for con excepción de
exception excepción *f*
excess exceso
excited agitado
exercise ejercicio
to exercise ejercer, hacer los ejercicios
to exist existir
expense gasto
to experience experimentar
explanation explicación *f*
to express expresar
to extract extraer
extraction extracción *f*
extremity extremidad *f*
eye ojo
eyeball globo del ojo
eyebrow ceja
eyeglasses anteojos *m pl*, espejuelos *m pl*, gafas *f pl*
eyelash pestaña
eyelid párpado
eyetooth colmillo

F

face cara
to face enfrentar(se) con
factor factor *m*
factory fábrica
to faint desmayarse
to fall caer(se); **to — asleep** dormirse
false teeth dentadura postiza
familiar *a* familiar
family familia
fat gordo
father padre *m*, papá *m*
favor favor *m*
fear miedo
February febrero
to feed alimentar, dar de comer
fertile fértil
fetus feto
fever calentura, fiebre *f;* **hay — ** fiebre de heno; **rheumatic — ** fiebre reumática; **scarlet — ** escarlatina; **yellow — ** fiebre amarilla
few pocos, -as
fibroma fibroma *m*
to fill llenar
filling empaste *m;* **to do a — ** empastar
finally por fin
to find encontrar, hallar; **to — out** averiguar
finger dedo; **index — ** dedo índice; **little — ** dedo meñique; **middle — ** dedo medio; **ring — ** dedo anular
to finish acabar, terminar
first primero
fish pescado
fist puño; **to make a — ** hacer un puño
to fix arreglar
flexible flexible
floor piso

flu influenza
fluid fluido
to fly volar
food alimento, comida
foolishness tontería
foot pie
for para; por
forceps forceps *m*
forehead frente *f*
to forget olvidar(se) de
form forma; formulario
formula fórmula
to fracture fracturar
free gratis
frequency frecuencia
frequently con frecuencia, frecuentemente
Friday viernes *m*
friend amigo, -a
frightened asustado
from de; desde
in front of enfrente de
fruit fruta
full lleno
to have fun divertirse
function función *f*

G

gallbladder vesícula biliar
gallstone cálculo biliar, piedra biliar
gangrene gangrena
to gargle hacer gárgaras
gargling gárgara
gas gas *m*
gastritis gastritis *m*
gastrointestinal gastrointestinal
gelatin gelatina
genital organs órganos genitales *m pl*
to get up levantarse
gift regalo
girl muchacha
girlfriend novia
to give dar; **— an injection** poner una inyección
glass vaso

glaucoma glaucoma *m*
to go ir(se)
gonorrhea gonorrea
good bueno
goodbye adiós
to grab agarrar(se) de
gradual gradual
grandfather abuelo
grandmother abuela
grapefruit toronja
grease grasa
greasy grasoso
greens verduras *f pl*
groin empeine *m*
gums encías
gynecologist ginecólogo, -a

H
habit hábito
hair cabello, pelo
half medio
to hallucinate alucinar
ham jamón *m*
hamburger hamburguesa
hand mano *f;* **back of the
— ** dorso de la mano
handsome guapo
to happen pasar, suceder
happy alegre
hard duro
harm daño; **to — oneself**
hacerse daño, dañarse
to have tener
head cabeza
headache dolor de cabeza
m, jaqueca
health salud *f*
hearing oído
heart corazón *m*
heat calor *m*
heating pad almohadilla
eléctrica
heel talón *m*
help ayuda
to help ayudar
hemorrhage hemorragia
hemorrhoids almorranas,
hemorroides *m pl*

hepatitis hepatitis *f*
here aquí
heroin heroína
high alto
hip cadera
hoarseness ronquera
to hold onto agarrar(se) de
to hope esperar
hospital hospital *m*
to hospitalize hospitalizar
hot caliente; **to be —** tener
calor
hour hora
house casa
housewife ama de casa
how? ¿cómo?; **how many?**
¿cuántos, -as?; **how much?**
¿cuánto?
hunger hambre *f*
to be hungry tener hambre
to hurt oneself dañarse,
hacerse daño
husband esposo, marido
hyperactive hiperactivo
hysterectomy histerectomía

I
ice cream helado
idea idea
immunization
inmunización *f*
to immunize inmunizar
impacted impactado
impatient impaciente
impediment impedimento
to impel impulsar
impertinent impertinente
impetigo impétigo
important importante
in en; dentro, dentro de
incisive incisivo
incisor incisivo
to include incluir
incompetent incompetente
incomprehensible
incomprensible
incubator incubadora
to indicate indicar

indigestion indigestión *f*
infant criatura; nene, nena
inferior inferior
inflamed inflamado
inflammation inflamación *f*
inflexible inflexible
influenza influenza
information información *f*
to inhale aspirar, inhalar
to inject inyectar
injection inyección *f*
to be injured lesionarse
injury herida, lesión *f*
ink tinta
to inoculate inocular
insane loco
to insert insertar, meter
inside of dentro de
instep empeine *m*
institution institución *f*
instruction instrucción *f*
insulin insulina
intelligent inteligente
to intend to pensar + *inf.*
interested interesado; **to be
— in** estar interesado en
intestine intestino
intravenous intravenoso;
— injection inyección
intravenosa *f*
to investigate investigar
iodine yodo
iron hierro
irregular irregular
irresponsible irresponsable
to irritate irritar
irritated irritado
irritation irritación *f*

J
January enero
jaw mandíbula, quijada
joint articulación *f*
juice jugo; **grapefruit —**
jugo de toronja; **orange —**
jugo de china, jugo de
naranja; **tomato —** jugo
de tomate
July julio

K

kidney riñón *m;* **— stone** piedra nefrítica
kind *a* amable; *n* tipo, clase de
kitchen cocina
knee rodilla
knife cuchillo
knot nudo
to know conocer; saber
knowledge conocimiento
knuckle nudillo

L

label etiqueta
labor labor *f;* parto
laboratory laboratorio
lamb cordero
lame cojo
language idioma *m,* lengua
large grande
laryngitis laringitis *f*
last último
to last durar
late tarde
later después, luego, más tarde
to laugh (at) reírse (de)
law ley *f*
laxative laxante *m*
to learn aprender; **to — to** aprender a
least menos; **at —** por lo menos
to leave dejar, salir
left izquierdo; **to the —** a la izquierda
leg pierna
lemon limón *m*
to lend prestar
lens lente *m;* **contact —** lente de contacto
lesion lesión *f*
less menos
lesson lección *f*
letter carta
lettuce lechuga
leukemia leucemia

to lie mentir
to lie down acostar(se); **lying down** acostado
light luz *f;* **to turn off the — ** apagar la luz; **to turn on the —** encender la luz
likable simpático
like como
to like (to be pleasing to) gustar
limitation limitación *f*
limited limitado
line línea
liniment linimento
link vínculo
lip labio
liquid líquido
to live vivir
liver hígado
lobster langosta
to look at mirar
to look for buscar
loop lazo
to lose perder; **— consciousness** perder el conocimiento
lump chichón *m*
lunch almuerzo; **to have —** almorzar
lung pulmón *m*

M

machine máquina; **ultrasonic —** máquina ultrasónica
mailman cartero
to make hacer
malaria malaria, paludismo
to malfunction funcionar mal
malignant maligno
malnutrition desnutrición *f*
mammography mamografía
man hombre *m*
manner manera; **in this —** de esta manera
many muchos
March marzo

margarine margarina
marijuana marihuana
married casado
massage masaje *m*
mastectomy mastectomía
maternity maternidad *f*
May mayo
maybe quizá, quizás
mayonnaise mayonesa
measles sarampión *m;* **German —** rubéola
to measure medir
meat carne *f*
mechanic mecánico
medication medicamento
medicine medicina
member miembro
meningitis meningitis *f*
menstruation menstruación *f*
method método; **birth control —** método anticonceptivo; **rhythm —** método de ritmo
mescaline mescalina
middle medio
midnight medianoche *f*
midwife partera
migraine migraña
milk leche; **— of magnesia** leche de magnesia
miscarriage aborto accidental
moist húmedo
molar muela
moment momento
Monday lunes *m*
money dinero
month mes *m*
more más; **— or less** más o menos
morning mañana; **— sickness** náuseas del embarazo, vómitos del embarazo
mother madre *f,* mamá
mouth boca; **roof of the —** cielo de la boca
to move mover

much mucho; **as —, so —**
tanto
mumps paperas *f pl*
mushroom hongo

N
nail uña
name nombre *m*
to be named llamarse
nape nuca
narcotic narcótico
nausea náuseas *f pl*
navel ombligo
necessary necesario
necessity necesidad *f*
neck cuello
to need necesitar
neighbor vecino
neither tampoco
nerve nervio; **to deaden
the —** adormecer el nervio
nervous agitado, nervioso;
— shock choque
nervioso *m*
neurologist neurólogo, -a
to neutralize neutralizar
nevertheless sin embargo
newspaper periódico
next próximo
night noche *f;* **last —**
anoche
nightmare pesadilla
nipple pezón *m; (on baby's
bottle)* pezón de biberón *m*
no no
no one nadie
noise ruido
none ninguno, -a
noon mediodía *m;* **at —** al
mediodía
normal normal
nose nariz *f;* **stuffed —**
nariz tupida, nariz tapada
nostrils fosas nasales *f pl*
not no
nothing nada
to notice notar
to notify notificar

November noviembre *m*
now ahora; **right —** ahora
mismo
number número
nurse enfermero, -a
nutrition nutrición *f*

O
obstetrician obstétrico, -a
obstetrics obstetricia
to obtain conseguir
obvious obvio
occupied ocupado
to occur ocurrir
October octubre *m*
of de
to offer ofrecer
office consultorio, oficina
official oficial
often a menudo
oil aceite *m*
ointment ungüento
old anciano, viejo
older mayor; **oldest** el/la
mayor
omelette tortilla
on en, encima de, sobre
onion cebolla
open abierto
to open abrir
to operate operar
operation operación *f*
ophthalmologist
oftalmólogo, -a
opinion opinión *f*
optician óptico
optometrist optometrista *mf*
oral oral
orange naranja
order *(harmony)* orden *m;*
order *(command)* orden *f*
to order mandar
orderly asistente *m*
organ órgano
orthopedist ortopédico, -a
other otro
ovary ovario
over sobre
overdose dosis excesiva *f*

to owe deber
oxygen oxígeno
oyster ostra

P
package paquete *m*
pain dolor *m;* **to be in —**
tener dolor; **labor —s**
dolores del parto
pair par *m;* **a — of** un par
de
pajamas pijamas *f pl*
palate paladar *m*
pale pálido
palm of the hand palma de
la mano
palpitation palpitación *f*
pancreas páncreas *m*
parallel bars barras
paralelas *f pl*
paralysis parálisis *m*
paralyzed paralizado
to pardon perdonar
parents padres *m pl*
part parte *f*
to participate participar
particular particular
to pass pasar
patella rótula
patience paciencia *f*
patient paciente *mf*
to pay pagar
pea guisante *m*
peach melocotón *m*
peanut butter crema de
cacahuete
pear pera
pediatrician pediatra *mf*
pelvis pelvis *f*
pen pluma
pencil lápiz *m*
to penetrate penetrar
penetrating penetrante
penicillin penicilina
penis pene *m*
pepper pimienta
period período; **menstrual
—** regla
permission permiso

to permit   permitir
personal   personal
pharmacist   farmacéutico
pharmacy   farmacia
phlegm   flema
physical   físico; **— exam**
   reconocimiento médico;
   — therapist   terapista
   físico *mf;* **— therapy**
   fisioterapia, terapia física
physician   médico
to pick up   recoger
pickle   pepinillo
picture   foto *f;* **to take —s**
   sacar fotos
pie   pastel *m*
piles   almorranas *f pl*
pill   pastilla, píldora;
   sleeping —   píldora para
   dormir
pillow   almohada
pipe   tubo
pistol   pistola
pity   lástima
pleasant   agradable
plum   ciruela
pneumonia   pulmonía
point   punto
poison   veneno
to be poisoned   envenenarse
police   policía
policeman   policía *m*
poliomyelitis   poliomielitis *f*
pork   puerco
possible   posible
possibly   posiblemente
potato   papa; **baked —**
   papa asada; **fried —**   papa
   frita
practice   práctica
to prefer   preferir
preferable   preferible
preferably   preferiblemente
pregnancy   embarazo
pregnancy test   prueba del
   embarazo
pregnant   embarazada,
   encinta, preñada; **to**
   become —   embarazarse

to prepare   preparar
to prescribe   recetar
prescription   receta
to press   apretar
pressure   presión *f;* **blood**
   —   presión arterial, presión
   sanguínea; **high blood —**
   presión alta; **low blood —**
   presión baja; **to take the**
   blood —   tomar la presión
pretty   lindo
priest   cura *m*
private   privado
problem   problema *m*
procedure   procedimiento
to produce   producir
profession   profesión *f*
professor   profesor, -a
profoundly   profundamente
prognosis   pronóstico
prophylatic   profiláctico
to protect   proteger
protection   protección *f*
protein   proteína
prune   ciruela pasa
psychiatrist   psiquíatra *mf*
psychiatry   psiquiatría
psychologist   psicólogo, -a
pudding   pudín *m*
to pull   tirar (de)
pulse   pulso; **to take the —**
   registrar el pulso
pupil   pupila
to push   empujar
to put   poner
(intravenous) pyelogram
   pielograma intravenoso *m*
pyorrhea   piorrea

Q

quantity   cantidad *f*
question   pregunta; **to ask a**
   —   hacer una pregunta
quickly   rápidamente
quiet   quieto

R

radioactive   radioactivo;
   — material   materia

radioactiva; **— substance**
   substancia radioactiva
radish   rábano
to raise   levantar; **to —**
   oneself, to get up
   levantarse
rape   violación *f*
to rape   violar
rash   salpullido
to read   leer
reading   lectura
ready   listo
reality   realidad *f;* **in —**   en
   realidad
really   de veras, realmente
reason   razón *f*
to receive   recibir
receptacle   vasija
receptionist   recepcionista
   mf
to recuperate   recuperar
relative   familiar *mf,*
   pariente, -a
relatively   relativamente
to relax   relajar(se)
to relieve   aliviar
to remain   quedar(se)
to remember   recordar,
   acordarse (de)
to remove   quitar(se)
to require   requerir
resistance   resistencia
to resort to   recurrir (a)
respiration   respiración *f;*
   artificial —   respiración
   artificial
respiratory   respiratorio
to respond   responder
responsibility
   responsabilidad *f*
responsible   responsable
rest   descanso
to rest   descansar
restless   inquieto
result   resultado
to resuscitate   resucitar
(mouth-to-mouth)
   resuscitation   respiración
   boca a boca

(mentally) retarded
atrasado mentalmente
to return volver
rib costilla
rice arroz *m*
rich rico
rickets raquitis *m*
right derecho; **to the —** a
la derecha; **to be —** tener
razón
ring anillo
to rinse enjuagar(se)
risk riesgo
roast beef rosbif *m*
room cuarto, sala; **double**
— cuarto doble; **private**
— cuarto privado;
recovery — sala de
recuperación
root raíz *f*
to run correr

S
saccharin sacarina
sad triste
safely con seguridad
safety seguridad *f*
saliva saliva
salmon salmón *m*
salt sal *f*
same mismo; **the —** lo
mismo
sardine sardina
to say decir
scalp cuero cabelludo
school escuela
to scratch (oneself)
rascar(se)
seasick mareado
to see ver
seldom pocas veces
to sell vender
sensation sensación *f*
separated separado
serious grave; serio
to serve servir
service servicio
set conjunto
severe severo

sexual sexual; **— relations**
relaciones sexuales *f pl*
sharp agudo
shellfish mariscos *m pl*
shield escudo
shin espinilla
shirt camisa
shoe zapato
shopkeeper dependiente, -a
short bajo
should deber
shoulder hombro; **— blade**
escápula, omóplato
to show mostrar
shower ducha
shrimp camarones *m pl*
sick enfermo; **to become**
— enfermarse
sickness enfermedad *f*
side lado
side effects efectos
secundarios
sight vista
sign señal *f*
to sign firmar
to signal señalar
since desde; ya que
single soltero
sister hermana
sister-in-law cuñada
size tamaño
skeleton esqueleto
skin piel *f*
skinny flaco, delgado
skull cráneo
to sleep dormir; **to fall —**
dormirse
sleeping durmiendo
slender delgado, flaco
slight leve
sling cabestrillo; **to put in a**
— poner en cabestrillo
slipper zapatilla
slowly despacio
smallpox viruela
smart listo
to smoke fumar
to sneeze estornudar
so así

soap jabón *m*
sober sobrio
soda soda
sole of the foot planta del
pie
solid sólido
solution solución *f*
some algunos, -as
something algo
son hijo
son-in-law yerno
soon pronto; **as — as**
possible lo más pronto
posible
Spanish español
to speak hablar
special especial
specialist especialista *mf*
to specialize
especializar(se)
specific específico
sperm esperma
spice especia
spinach espinaca
spiral espiral *f*
to spit escupir
spleen bazo, esplín *m*
spoon cuchara
spoonful cucharada
sprain torcedura
to sprain torcer
to squeeze apretar
to stab apuñalar
to stagger tambalear
stairs escalera; **downstairs**
escalera abajo; **upstairs**
escalera arriba
to stand parar(se), poner(se)
de pie
standing parado, de pie
state estado; **— of health**
estado de salud
to stay quedar(se)
sterilization esterilización *f*
to sterilize esterilizar
still todavía; quieto
stomach estómago; **(to lie)**
on one's — boca abajo
stone cálculo, piedra

to stop dejar
straight recto
strained colado
strange extraño
strawberry fresa
street calle *f*
strenuous estrenuo
stretcher camilla; **to carry on a —** llevar en camilla; **stretcher-bearer** camillero
strong fuerte
to study estudiar
such tal
to suffer from padecer
sufficient bastante, suficiente
to suffocate ahogar(se)
sugar azúcar *m*
suicide suicidio; **to attempt —** atentar el suicidio
suitcase maleta
Sunday domingo
sunglasses gafas de sol *f pl*
sure cierto, seguro
surgeon cirujano, -a
surgery cirugía
to suspect sospechar
to swallow tragar
swelling hinchazón *m*
syrup jarabe *m*
system sistema *m;* **circulatory —** sistema circulatorio; **digestive —** sistema digestivo; **nervous —** sistema nervioso; **respiratory —** sistema respiratorio

T
table mesa
tablet tableta
to take tomar; **— charge of** encargarse de; **— precautions** precaucionar(se)
talcum talco
to talk hablar
tall alto
tea té *m*

teacher maestro, -a
technician técnico
telephone teléfono; **— call** llamada telefónica
television televisión *f*
to tell decir
temperature temperatura
test examen *m,* prueba
to test probar
testicle testículo
tetanus tétano
thank you gracias
that que
then entonces, luego
therapist terapeuta, terapista *mf*
therapy terapia
there is, there are hay
thigh muslo
thin delgado, flaco
thing cosa
to think pensar; **— about** pensar en
thorax tórax *m*
throat garganta
to throw echar; **to — away** botar
thumb pulgar *m,* dedo pulgar
Thursday jueves *m*
time hora; tiempo, vez; **at the same —** al mismo tiempo; **at —s** a veces; **for a long —** por mucho tiempo; **many —s** muchas veces; **one —** una vez; **sometimes** a veces
tincture of iodine tinta de yodo
tired cansado; **to become —** cansarse
to a
today hoy
toe dedo del pie
tolerant tolerante
tomato tomate *m*
tomorrow mañana; **the day after —** pasado mañana
tongue lengua
tonsils amígdalas *f pl*

too también; **— many** demasiados, -as; **— much** demasiado
tooth diente *m;* **decayed —** diente cariado; **false teeth** dentadura postiza; **milk —** diente de leche; **to fill a —** empastar
toothbrush cepillo de dientes
to touch tocar
tourniquet torniquete *m*
toward hacia
towel toalla
toxemia toxemia
traditional tradicional
tranquilizer calmante *m,* tranquilizante *m*
to transmit transmitir
treatment tratamiento
truly de veras
truth verdad *f*
to try probar; **to — to** tratar de
tubal ligation ligadura de los tubos
tube tubo
tuberculosis tuberculosis *f*
Tuesday martes *m*
tumor tumor *m*
tuna atún *m*
turn turno
to turn doblar; torcer
twin gemelo
to twist torcer
type tipo, clase de
typhoid tifoidea

U
ugly feo
ulcer úlcera
ultrasound transmitter transmisor ultrasonido *m*
umbilical cord cordón umbilical *m*
uncle tío
uncomfortable incómodo
underneath abajo, debajo de

to understand comprender
underwear ropa interior
unguent ungüento
unmarried soltero
unpleasant antipático
until hasta
up arriba
upstairs escalera arriba
urinalysis urinálisis *m*,
análisis de la orina *m*
urine orina
to use usar
useless inútil
uterus útero

V

vagina vagina
vaginal cream crema
vaginal
varied variado
vasectomy vasectomía
veal ternera
vegetable legumbre *f*,
vegetal *m*
vertebral column columna
vertebral
very muy
victim víctima
vinegar vinagre *m*
to violate violar
virus virus *m*
vision visión *f*, vista; **to
have good —** tener
buena vista
visit visita
to visit visitar
vitamin vitamina
vomit vómito
to vomit vomitar

W

waist cintura
to wait esperar

waiter camarero
waiting room sala de
espera
waitress camarera
to wake up despertar(se)
to walk caminar
to want desear, querer
ward cuarto múltiple
warm caliente
to warn avisar
to wash (oneself) lavar(se)
washbasin lavabo
to watch over velar
water agua; **bag of —s**
bolsa de aguas; **mineral —**
agua mineral
weak débil
Wednesday miércoles *m*
to weigh pesar
weight peso; **to gain —**
aumentar de peso; **to lose
—** perder peso
(you're) welcome de nada,
no hay de qué
well bien
well-being bienestar *m*
wet mojado
what que; **what?** ¿qué?,
¿cuál?
when cuando; **when?**
¿cuándo?
where donde; **where?**
¿dónde?; **to where?** ¿a
dónde?
which? ¿cuál?
while mientras
white blanco
who, whom quien, quienes;
who?, whom? ¿quién?,
¿quiénes?
whooping cough tos
ferina *f*
why? ¿por qué?

widow viuda
widower viudo
wife esposa, mujer
to win ganar
window ventana
wine vino
wisdom tooth muela del
juicio
to wish querer
with con
withdrawal retirada
within por dentro
woman mujer
womb matriz *f*, vientre *m*
work empleo, trabajo
to work trabajar
worker trabajador, -a
worried preocupado
to worry preocupar(se)
worse peor
to worsen empeorar
wrist muñeca
to write escribir

X

X-ray radiografía, rayos X;
to take an — hacer una
radiografía

Y

year año; **last —** el año
pasado
yesterday ayer; **the day
before —** anteayer
yet todavía, aún
yolk yema (de huevo)
young joven *mf*; **younger**
menor; **youngest** el/la
menor
youth juventud *f*

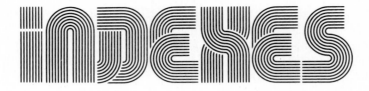

Index of Grammatical and Structural Items

Index of Medical Vocabulary

B
C
D
E
F 4
G 5
H 6
I 7
J 8
9